T0344262

Healing in Urology

Clinical Guidebook to Herbal and Alternative Therapies

Healing in Urology

Clinical Guidebook to Herbal and Alternative Therapies

Editors

Bilal Chughtai
Weill Cornell Medical College, USA

Amy Stein
Beyond Basics Physical Therapy, LLC, USA

Geo Espinosa
New York University Medical Center, USA

World Scientific

NEW JERSEY · LONDON · SINGAPORE · BEIJING · SHANGHAI · HONG KONG · TAIPEI · CHENNAI · TOKYO

Published by

World Scientific Publishing Co. Pte. Ltd.

5 Toh Tuck Link, Singapore 596224

USA office: 27 Warren Street, Suite 401-402, Hackensack, NJ 07601

UK office: 57 Shelton Street, Covent Garden, London WC2H 9HE

Library of Congress Cataloging-in-Publication Data
Names: Chughtai, Bilal, editor.
Title: Healing in urology : clinical guidebook to herbal and alternative therapies /
   [edited by] Bilal Chughtai.
Description: New Jersey : World Scientific, 2016. | Includes bibliographical references.
Identifiers: LCCN 2016000018 | ISBN 9789814719087 (hc : alk. paper)
Subjects: | MESH: Urologic Diseases--therapy | Complementary Therapies |
   Psychotherapy
Classification: LCC RC900.5 | NLM WJ 166 | DDC 616.6/06--dc23
LC record available at http://lccn.loc.gov/2016000018

British Library Cataloguing-in-Publication Data
A catalogue record for this book is available from the British Library.

Copyright © 2017 by World Scientific Publishing Co. Pte. Ltd.

All rights reserved. This book, or parts thereof, may not be reproduced in any form or by any means, electronic or mechanical, including photocopying, recording or any information storage and retrieval system now known or to be invented, without written permission from the publisher.

For photocopying of material in this volume, please pay a copying fee through the Copyright Clearance Center, Inc., 222 Rosewood Drive, Danvers, MA 01923, USA. In this case permission to photocopy is not required from the publisher.

Desk Editors: Suraj Kumar/Joy Quek

Typeset by Stallion Press
Email: enquiries@stallionpress.com

Printed in Singapore

Contents

About the Editors   vii

Disclaimer   ix

Chapter 1   Introduction   1
             Dominique Thomas, Claire Dunphy
             and Bilal Chughtai

Chapter 2   Eastern Herbal Medicine   5
             Mindy Pickard

Chapter 3   Western Herbal Medicine   19
             Eric Yarnell

Chapter 4   Naturopathy   45
             Geo Espinosa and Ralph Esposito Jr

Chapter 5   Functional Nutrition for Pelvic Health   91
             Jessica Drummond

Chapter 6   Acupuncture   109
             Jillian Capodice

Chapter 7   Physical Therapy Evaluation and Manual
             Therapy Treatment Strategies for Pelvic
             and Urologic Disorders   129
             *Jennafer Vande Vegte, Bridgid Ellingson
             and Amy Stein*

Chapter 8   Adjunct Modalities for Physical Therapy   165
             *Lila Bartkowski-Abbate, Allison Ariail
             and Andrea Wood*

Chapter 9   Yoga   185
             Dustienne Miller

Chapter 10   Osteopathy for Urologic and Pelvic Health   209
             Daniel Lopez

Chapter 11   Cognitive Behavioral Therapy   223
             Alexandra Milspaw

Chapter 12   Psychodynamic Psychotherapy   243
             Jennifer Schimmel

Index   265

About the Editors

Bilal Chughtai, MD, is a urologist specializing in female urology and voiding dysfunction. He is appointed as an Assistant Professor in the departments of both Urology and Obstetrics and Gynecology at Weill Cornell Medicine-New York Presbyterian. Dr. Chughtai completed his undergraduate degree in Biology at New York University, then went on to complete medical school at the State University of New York at Stony Brook, and his residency at Albany Medical Center. He has completed a fellowship at both Weill Cornell Medicine and Memorial Sloan Kettering Cancer Center in Female Pelvic Medicine and Reconstructive Surgery and Voiding Dysfunction.

Dr. Chughtai is a leader in Female Pelvic Medicine and Reconstructive Surgery and Voiding Dysfunction, he has been an investigator in numerous clinical trials, translational, and outcomes research that include National Institute of Health and industry support. He is a reviewer for several prestigious journals such as Lancet, JAMA Surgery, European Urology, Journal of Urology, Urology as well as an editor for several urological journals. He has published over 100 peer-reviewed articles, authored chapters in several urologic texts, published two textbooks, and has presented numerous abstracts at national meetings.

Geo Espinosa, N.D., L.Ac, C.N.S., RH (AHG), is a renowned naturopathic and functional medicine doctor recognized as an authority in urology and men's health. Dr. Geo is the founder and director of the Integrative and Functional Urology Center at New York University Langone Medical Center (NYULMC) and lectures internationally on the application of integrative urology in clinical settings. He has been recognized as one of the top 10 Health Makers for Men's Health by sharecare.com created by Dr. Mehmet Oz and WebMD. Dr. Geo is the author of the popular book: *"Thrive, Don't Only Survive: Dr. Geo's Guide to Living Your Best Life Before & After Prostate Cancer."*

Amy Stein, DPT, is a leading expert and at the forefront of treating pelvic floor dysfunction, pelvic pain, women's health, and functional manual therapy for men, women, and children. She is the founder of, and a premier practitioner at Beyond Basics Physical Therapy in NYC. She is the author of *Heal Pelvic Pain*, an easy-read, self-help book and created a video called *Healing Pelvic and Abdominal Pain: The ultimate home program for patients and a guide for practitioners*. Amy is one of the founders of the Alliance for Pelvic Pain, a patient-oriented educational retreat, and she serves as the Vice President of the International Pelvic Pain Society.

Amy is an author in the medical textbooks, *Female Sexual Pain Disorders: Evaluation and Management* and *The Overactive Pelvic Floor*. She lectures internationally, is featured in the *Endo What?* documentary, and has been interviewed in media outlets ranging from the medical segments of popular TV shows, like Dr. Oz, ABC's 20/20, to such magazines as Elle, Prevention and More magazine and newspapers such as the New York Daily News. She is a member of ISSWSH, the NVA, ISSVD, ICA, and the APTA Women's Health section. Amy received her Masters in Physical Therapy from Nova Southeastern University in 1999, and her Doctorate in Physical Therapy in 2013.

Disclaimer

Although the author and publisher have made every effort to ensure that the information in this book was correct at press time, the author and publisher do not assume and hereby disclaim any liability to any party for any loss, damage, or disruption caused by errors or omissions, whether such errors or omissions result from negligence, accident, or any other cause.

This book is not intended as a substitute for the medical advice of physicians. The reader should regularly consult a physician in matters relating to his/her health and particularly with respect to any symptoms that may require diagnosis or medical attention.

Chapter 1

Introduction

**Dominique Thomas, Claire Dunphy and
Bilal Chughtai**

Weill Cornell Medical College, New York

Healing in Urology is a biography of medical practices. Healing addresses the experience of the health patron (patient) and the outcomes of different approaches to prevent recurrence of the illness. The burden of health treatment to alleviate the physical suffering of these health seekers is taxing on the body and on the pocket. In 2013, the United States spent more $2.9 trillion on health expenditures.[1] Because of this and other factors, the medical field has developed ways to improve health literacy for those with health concerns by broadening the scope of medical treatments to assess the use of alternative forms of healing.[2] An outcome of this has placed accountability on both the health professional and the health patron to take initiative toward innovation.[2-4]

Interestingly, "alternative" medicine in various parts of the world has been their norm for generations. These populations of people practiced medicine by performing sacred healing ceremonies, concocting health elixirs and using forms of pray and devotion to deities to eradicate the body of illness.[2,5] A common practice was the use of herbal remedies prescribed by a health shaman. This was to provide the sufferer with ways to not only focus on the illness, but to open the body up to positive energy.[5,6] The use of herbal medicines in other countries has been integrated into their formal method of medical training in other countries.[2]

In the United States, alternative forms of medicine have been utilized in a different manner than traditional healing ceremonies. This alternative method can be complementary to the use of a herbal supplement to treat infection vs. using a course of antibiotics.[7] Despite embracing the use of herbal supplementations, the efficacy utilizing alternative methods to treat illness has not been rigorously validated like more traditional methods.[8] The medical evidence of medical alternatives is still in its infancy. We need to produce more research to comprehend how different practices are being integrated into contemporary treatment methods. Research conducted by scientists suggests there is a growing demand to investigate alternative healing practices to treat medical problems in modern medicine.[8] The goal is to exercise knowledge in understanding the benefits of these complementary medicines and discovering which parts of the mind and body are affected.

In medicine, urological disorders are of special interest when researching the use of alternative medicines because of the non-discriminatory nature of these diseases to affect all people[9]; thus healing in urology can be universal. Physicians can adopt different healing approaches such as manual therapy to the use of yoga to treat the health patron's symptoms. Because of their simplicity, we can utilize the complementarity of similar and disparate urological approaches. This manual will explore a myriad of therapies, behavioral changes and utilization of herbal regiments to address the incidence of disease to alleviate the symptoms experienced by the health patron. Each chapter will tackle a remedy, demonstrating its effectiveness through research data and the personal narratives from healthcare professionals. Furthermore, as you navigate through the different approaches addressing urological disorders, you'll notice some focus on the mind specifically while others on the body. Some philosophies teach the student that the mind has the ability to heal the body by harnessing positive energy,[10] while others focus on manipulating the body. Students are taught to nourish the body with healthy food and maintain a balanced lifestyle by respecting the body through exercise. These medical treatments provide a holistic perspective on "patient" healing.

The goal of this book is to provide healthcare professionals with alternative methods to treating urological disorders, involve health patrons in the treatment by making these practices patient-centered, and demonstrate patient and physician can build a foundation of alternative methods alongside standard of care to ensure the patient feels comfort in their "normal". We wrote this book to enlighten healthcare professionals in urology about the many tools we can equip ourselves with when treating those with these illnesses, sicknesses, and diseases. By integrating our knowledge and collaborating with other fields we can make treatment and healing more encompassing and efficient. The beauty of these practices is the agelessness of their use.

We want to get people to think about ways to care for the patient and for the body by utilizing things that are readily available on a daily basis, that are natural. We can always wait for the next drug or surgery, but what can we do in the present to improve the course of illness. We challenge you, the health promoter, next time you are required to heal, you exercise openness to not only addressing the health concern, but also blessing the health patron with their own tools to be active in the treatment acquisition. With this knowledge, it is our hope healthcare professionals will determine ways of integrating these approaches into their already established standard of care routines.

References

1. National Center for Health Statistics. Health, United States, 2014: With Special Feature on Adults Aged 55–64. Hyattsville, MD; 2015.
2. Mishra SR, Neupane D and Kallestrup P. Integrating complementary and alternative medicine into conventional health care system in developing countries: an example of Amchi. *J Evid Based Complementary Altern Med.* 2015;20:76–79.
3. Zuger A. Talking to patients in the 21st century. *JAMA.* 2013;309: 2384–2385.
4. Leshner AI. Beyond the teachable moment. *JAMA.* 2007;298: 1326–1328.
5. Bussmann RW. The globalization of traditional medicine in northern peru: from shamanism to molecules. *Evid Based Complement Alternat Med.* 2013;2013:291903.
6. Hewson P, Rowold J, Sichler C and Walter W. Are healing ceremonies useful for enhancing quality of life? *J Altern Complement Med.* 2014;20:713–717.
7. Khan MA, Singh M, Khan MS, Ahmad W, Najmi AK and Ahmad S. Alternative approach for mitigation of doxorubicin-induced cardiotoxicity using herbal agents. *Curr Clin Pharmacol.* 2014;9: 288–297.
8. Welliver D. Pharmacologic matters of herbal supplements. *Gastroenterol Nurs.* 2011;34:321–322.
9. Markland AD, Thompson IM, Ankerst DP, Higgins B and Kraus SR. Lack of disparity in lower urinary tract symptom severity between community-dwelling non-Hispanic white, Mexican-American, and African-American men. *Urology.* 2007;69:697–702.
10. Delany C, Miller KJ, El-Ansary D, Remedios L, Hosseini A and McLeod S. Replacing stressful challenges with positive coping strategies: a resilience program for clinical placement learning. *Adv Health Sci Educ Theory Pract.* 2015;20:1303–1324.

Chapter 2

Eastern Herbal Medicine

Mindy Pickard

Three Treasures Acupuncture, PC New York, NY 10002

Eastern Herbal Medicine offers natural and effective solutions to many pelvic and urological conditions for men and women. An overview of Eastern Herbal medicine theory and diagnostics is discussed, followed by herbal recommendations for many conditions such as constipation, pelvic pain, disorders of the libido and orgasm, benign prostatic hyperplasia, incontinence, UTI, Interstitial cystitis/painful bladder syndrome (IC/PBS) and kidney stones. The use of these formulas is based on historical and clinical experience.

Introduction to Chinese Herbal Medicine

Chinese Herbal Medicine has been practiced in China for more than 2,000 years. About 1,800 years ago, Chang Chung-Ching compiled a compendium called the *Shang Han Lun* or "Treatise on Febrile Diseases". This work is considered the first text of Chinese Medicine and is the basis for *Kanpo*, the Japanese system of Chinese Herbal Medicine that I practice.

Kanpo primarily comprises ancient, classic formulas. *Kanpo* means "the way of the *Han*" and refers to the herbal medicine that was brought to Japan during the Sui and Tang dynasties. The classic formulas tend to be simpler than modern formulas, comprising five to eight different herbs for the most part. "*Kanpo* is an ancient system, faithful to herbal formulas used for centuries throughout the Orient, but also a modern system, withstanding the scrutiny of cutting-edge scientific technique."[1]

In addition to the *Shang Han Lun*, there is another ancient text, the *Chin Kuei Yao Lueh* or "Prescriptions from the Golden Chamber." According to scholars, these two texts were originally one book, the *Shang Han Tsu-Ping Lun* or "Annotated Treatise on Febrile Diseases."

Most formulas in use today are either exactly the same as they were prescribed in these ancient texts or derived from these earliest formulas to create modern formulas.

The **dosing** of herbal formulas in *Kanpo* is also based on historical and clinical efficacy. As a rule of thumb, for granulated formulas I prescribe 2 g per dose, three times a day for adults. With patent medicines, the dosing can be variable and based on the experience of the practitioner.

Chinese Herbal Theory

Yin yang theory is the underlying basis of all Chinese philosophy and medical theory. The concept is very ancient and is thought to have been devised more than 5,000 years ago. *Yin* is characterized by dark, deep, submerged, passive, and weak things. *Yang* is described as light, superficial, ascending, active, positive, and strong.[2]

All disease is considered as an imbalance of *yin and yang* according to Chinese medical theory. Simplistically stated, if a person is too *yin*, give *yang* tonics, and vice versa, if a person is too *yang*, give *yin* tonics.

Yin yang theory can be further refined by differentiating whether the site of the disease is **interior** or **surface**; whether the nature of the disease is **fever** or **chill**, and whether the disease presentation is **strong** or **weak**.

In the 18th century, another theory was established in Japan, called the **Qi, Blood, and Water** theory. *Qi* ("Chee") or, *Ki* in Japanese, is an unseen but vital substance that circulates in the body. Some translate the word as energy or life force. *Qi* is considered *yang*, energetically speaking. Blood in Chinese medicine is considered *yin* and is defined as both the blood that circulates in our body, and also the bodily fluids. This theory maintains that as long as there is balance between *Qi*, blood, and fluids, there will be no disease. When one of these is blocked or overpowers the other two, there is disharmony. "Successful Chinese herbal therapy consists of correcting all excesses, deficiencies, and stagnations of *Qi*, blood, and water".[2]

Herbal formulas can also be classified according to the *Qi*, blood, and fluids theory. *Qi* stagnation is treated with *Qi* regulating formulas. Water stagnation is usually the same as saying dampness or one could have dampness in one area and dryness in the rest of the body. This is usually treated with fluid regulating formulas. Lastly, blood disharmony, either deficiency or stagnation, is treated with blood regulating formulas.

Blood stagnation, called **Oketsu** in Japanese medicine, is an important diagnostic tool in *Kanpo*. It is found by palpating the abdomen below and diagonally to the side of the navel. If these points bring about a wince on the part of the patient when palpated, then *Oketsu* is suspected and treated first before anything else. "Like a clog in a drainage pipe, stagnant blood can create all kinds of problems in the housekeeping of the body."[1] One of the causes of *Oketsu* on a microlevel is chronic inflammation; the small microcirculation blood vessels are damaged due to inflammation and create blockage, where the blood pools and occludes. "The area by the left *iliac fossa* in a woman is known to be equivalent to the hypersensitive zone which refers to the left ovary and uterine duct; the area in the right *ileac fossa* is often associated with the ileocecal valve, appendix, and ascending colon."[3]

The **nature** of the herbal formula is also paramount when determining which remedy to utilize. There are primarily 10 different types of formulas: warming, cooling, tonifying, purgative, drying, moistening, ascending, descending, dispersing, and contracting. Each herbal category is used to treat the opposite conformation found in the person. For example, a person suffering from a dry cough would be given a formula with a moistening nature. Formulas can also have more than one nature, i.e. they can have many properties depending on the separate herbs. It is the "complex intermingling of the numerous properties" of the herbs that creates the overall nature of the formula.[2]

Diagnostic Procedures

Chinese herbal medicine is ancient medicine. It was created thousands of years before there were any blood tests, X-rays or c-scans. The ancient herbalist had to rely on their senses to determine the diagnosis — looking, listening and smelling, questioning and touching. Today, this process is called the *Four Examinations* and remains the basis for all modern Asian medicine.

The first important sense for the diagnostician is visual. How does the patient present? How do their eyes, skin, body shape look? How does their tongue present? The second is listening. What does the patient sound like? What is the timbre of their voice? What about their breathing — is it labored or raspy? And, most importantly, what do they report about their condition? How do they describe it? The third sense is smell. How a patient smells was paramount to ancient diagnosis and different odors are attributable to different organ energetics in Chinese medicine.

The last sense is touch, palpation. All Chinese medicine incorporates pulse diagnosis, which has been elevated to an art form in modern practice. But it is primarily *Kanpo* medicine that relies on abdominal palpation as being the most paramount to the diagnostic process.

There are 14 abdominal conformations in *Kanpo*. Some are relatively easy to ascertain: like a tight rectus abdominis muscle, tight hypochondriac area or emptiness below the navel. Others are a bit harder to sensitize to as a practitioner. Each abdominal conformation is a blueprint, or a diagnostic hint if you will, to a group of herbal formulas that would be germane to the findings. For instance, a tightness under the ribs in the hypochondriac area usually points to the use of bupleurum-based formulas, whereas tight rectus abdominis muscles point to the use of cinnamon-based formulas.

Modern Research

Over the past 25 years, there has been a concerted effort made on the part of herbal manufacturers and herbal medicine doctors in China and Japan to systematically prove, from a modern research paradigm, that Chinese formulas work. The problem is that many research studies done in China and Japan are not translated into English. Additionally, many Western pharmaceutical companies are investigating the efficacy of Chinese herbs for development into new drugs.

Despite this lack of hard data in English, we as herbalists practicing in the West feel confident of our practices because Chinese herbal medicine has thousands of years of clinical efficacy behind it and very few side effects. "One of *Kanpo's* greatest advantages is its power to heal gently, without causing serious side effects."[1]

The greatest asset that *Kanpo* medicine has over pharmaceutical drugs is that it is a patient-centered medicine. It's not "one size fits all" paradigm like pharmaceutical drugs. "...this ancient system of herbal healing was designed to treat not diseases but people. The future may bring new bacteria, new viruses and new threats to health. But the gift of *Kanpo* lies in its ageless ability to improve the condition of the whole person."[1]

The Conditions

Clear *Oketsu* first!

Clinically, I have found that most pelvic pain patients suffer from either chronic constipation or IBS and most female patients suffer from menstrual irregularities as well. Many of these patients have a palpable blood stasis conformation (*Oketsu*). If there is a palpable blood stasis point, I try to clear the *Oketsu* first and usually start them on one of the following formulas:

- Cinnamon and Hoelen Combination (*Gui Zhi Fu Ling Tang*)
- Persica and Rhubarb Combination (left sided *Oketsu*) (*Tao He Cheng Qi Tang*)
- Rhubarb and Moutan Combination (right sided *Oketsu*) (*Da HuangMu Dan Pi Tang*)

Bowel/GI Dysfunction

Many Chinese herbalists start from the standing point of digestion. We feel that there will not be optimum health if the patient is not transporting and transforming their food well. Also, from a practical standpoint, if there are problems with the bowel, this is often affecting their other bodily systems as well.

After using a blood stasis formula to clear for *Oketsu* for a few weeks, I move to a more traditional constipation formula. There are several to choose from and the choice is dependent on many factors: heat or cold, strong or weak conformation, dry or not dry stool and body type.

The strong conformation formulas are as follows:

- Major Bupleurum Combination (*Da Chai Hu Tang*)
- Cimicifuga Combination (*I Zhu Tang*)
- Rhubarb and Licorice Combination (*Da Huang Gan Cao Tang*)
- Coptis and Rhubarb (*San Huang Xie Xin Tang*)
- Rhubarb and Mirabilitum (*Tiao Wei Cheng Qi Tang*)
- Persica and Rhubarb Combination (*Tao He Cheng Qi Tang*)
- Rhubarb and Moutan Combination (*Da Huang Mu Dan Pi Tang*)

For more moderate conformations, we use Minor Bupleurum Combination (*Xiao Chai Hu Tang*).

Those with weaker constitutions should consider the following formulas:

- Linum and Rhubarb Combination (*Jun Chang Tang*)
- Apricot and Linum Combination (*Ma Zhu Zhen Tang*)
- Major Zanthoxylum Combination plus Minor Cinnamon and Peony Combination (*Da Jian Zhong Tang* plus *Da Jian Zhong Tang*)
- Cinnamon, Peony, and Rhubarb Combination (*Gui Zhi Jia Shao Yao Da Huang Tang*)

Clinically, I use Cinnamon, Peony and Rhubarb Combination most frequently with pelvic pain and urologic patients that suffer from chronic constipation. Many of these patients have perennially tight abdominal muscles and this formula works to relax those muscles over time. I have found Major Zanthoxylum Combination, with or without the addition of Minor Cinnamon and Peony Combination, to be the most useful for IBS patients.

Other formulas that work well with IBS include:

- Cinnamon and Peony Combination (*Gui Zhi Shao Tang*)
- Cinnamon, Peony, and Rhubarb Combination (*Gui Zhi Jia Shao Yao Da Huang Tang*)

For stress-induced IBS, or for IBS that tends more toward diarrhea with an emotional component, I use:

- Bupleurum and Cinnamon Combination (*Chai Hu Gui Zhi Tang*)
- Lotus and Citrus Combination (Qi Pi Tang)
- Pinellia Combination (*Ban Xia Xie Xin Tang*)
- For IBS that tends more towards diarrhea I use: Ginseng and Ginger Combination (*Zhen Shen Tang*)
- Vitality Combination (*Zhen Wu Tang*)
- Cardamom and Fennel Combination (*An Zhong San*)
- Four or Six Major Herb Combinations (*Si/Lui Jun Zi Tang*)

Pelvic Pain

Many of my female pelvic pain patients suffer from vulvodynia, vestibulitis, clitoradynia and similar newly-coined conditions. Most of them also suffer from menstrual irregularities, such as amenorrhea, dysmenorrhea or menorrhagia. Since there is not any mention of the new diagnoses in the herbal literature, I first work with what I know. If the patient suffers from dysmenorrhea, I use the following formulas:

- Cinnamon and Hoelen Combination (*Gui Zhi Fu Ling Tang*)
- Persica and Rhubarb Combination (*Tao He Cheng Qi Tang*)
- Cinnamon and Persica Combination (*Zhe Chong Yin*)
- Dang Gui and Peony Combination (*Dang Gui Shao Yao San*)

If the woman suffers from Amenorrhea or light period or missed periods, I use the following:

- Dang Gui and Peony Combination (*Dang Gui Shao Yao San*)
- Dang Gui Four Combination Combination (*Si Wu Tang*)
- Bupleurum and Peony Combination (*Jia Wei Xiao Yao San*)

For menorrhagia or break through bleeding, I choose from the following:

- Dang Gui, Cinnamon and Peony Combination (*Dang Gui Jian Zhong Tang*)
- Cinnamon and Persica Combination (*Zhe Chong Yin*)
- Ginseng and Astragalus Combination (*Bu Zhong Yi Qi Tang*)
- Ginseng and Longan Combination (*Gui Pi Tang*)

For those pelvic pain conditions that are more a problem of cold or fluid imbalance in the lower abdomen, I use the following:

- Dang Gui and Peony Combination (*Dang Gui Shao Yao San*)
- Dang Gui, Evodia and Ginger Combination (*Dang Gui Wu Zhu Yu Sheng Jiang Tang*)
- Dang Gui and Evodia Combination (*Wen Jing Tang*)

Clinically, I have also found Cimicifuga Combination (*I Zhu Tang*) to be efficacious in cases of vulvar, vestibular, and clitoral pain. Traditionally, it is used for hemorrhoids, but I believe the same action that brings blood and nourishment to the hemorrhoids will also bring it to the genitals. And lastly, Peony and Licorice Combination (*Shao Yao Gan Cao Tang*) and its cousin formula Peony, Licorice and Aconite Combination (*Shao Yao Gan Cao Fu Zi Tang*) are good formulas to use for acute, spasmodic pain in the pelvic region. It acts quickly to relieve pain and congestion in the area.

Disorders of Libido and Disorders of Orgasm

While thinking about disorders of libido, we as practitioners have to peel the onion so to speak, to unravel what is causing the lowered libido, orgasm dysfunction, erectile disorder or ejaculation problems. Is it pain from sexual activity or orgasm or is it from aging and lowered hormones? If it is from pain, I follow the protocol above for pelvic pain disorders and try to improve those outcomes first.

If it is from lowered hormones which are often the result of the aging process, which in Chinese medicine, we attribute to lowered "kidney energy", or the kidney *Qi* not being firm, I use the following formulas:

- Rehmannia 6 (*Lui Wei Di Huang Wan*)
- Rehmannia 8 (*Ba Wei Di Huang Wan*)
- Lycium Formula (*Huan Shao Dan*)
- Cinnamon and Dragon Bone Combination (*Gui Zhi Jia Long Gu Mu Li Tang*)
- Bupleurum and Dragon Bone Combination (*Chai Hu Jia Long Gu Mu Li Tang*)
- Bupleurum Formula (*Yi Gan San*)
- Bupleurum, Cinnamon, and Ginger (*Chai Hu Gui Zhi Gan Jiang Tang*)
- Ginseng and Astragalus (*Bu Zhong Yi Qi Tang*)

Man's Treasure — this is not a *Kanpo* formula, but a patent formula from Seven Forests for which I have great results. I use it for men with low back pain, low libido, and urinary frequency.

Benign Prostatic Hyperplasia

Many men with prostate enlargement or BPH have *Oketsu*, signifying vascular constriction around the prostate. It is usually accompanied by severe pain, swelling, and constipation. For these patients, I start with one of the following blood stasis formulas:

- Cinnamon and Hoelen Combination (*Gui Zhi Fu Ling Tang*)
- Rhubarb and Moutan Combination (*Da Huang Mu Dan Pi Tang*)
- Persica and Rhubarb Combination (*Tao He Chen Qi Tang*)

Other men with BPH are suffering from the aging process and have "Kidney deficiency" from a Chinese medicine standpoint. Usually, these patients are tired, have low back pain and may have erectile dysfunction.

For these men, I choose:

- Rehmannia 6 or 8 (*Lui/Ba Wei Di Huang Wan*)

Either of these formulas can be combined with Cinnamon and Hoelen Combination when the patient suffers from pelvic/genital pain, blood stasis, back pain, and low libido. When there are inflammatory signs and symptoms, pressure on bladder, scanty urination use the following:

- Polyporus Combination (*Zhu Ling Tang*)

If there is inflammation and heat signs, such as dark scanty urine and itching in the genital region use the following:

- Gentiana Combination (*Long Dan Xie Gan Tang*)

Incontinence

Chinese herbal medicine does not distinguish between enuresis and polyuria. However, it does distinguish between stress and urge incontinence. For those patients that complain about urinary incontinence at night or during daytime naps, I prescribe the following formulas, which address the dysfunction of the tone of the abdominal muscles (either too tight from deficiency or lacking in tone):

- Minor Cinnamon and Peony Combination (*Xiao Jian Zhong Tang*)
- Rehmannia 8 Combination (*Ba Wei Di Huang Wan*)
- Lotus Seed Combination (*Qing Xin Lian Zi Yin*)
- Pueraria Combination (*Ge Gen Tang*)

For urge incontinence, where the patient does not have the sensitivity or lacks control or awareness of the urge, use Rehmannia 8 Combination.

For stress incontinence, consider the following:

- Minor Bupleurum Combination plus Minor Cinnamon and Peony Combination (*Xiao Chai Hu Tang plus Xiao Jian Zhong Tang*)

Urinary Tract Infection (UTI)

There are four primary formulas for combating a UTI in *Kanpo*. Choosing a formula depends on whether it is in the acute or chronic phase. For the acute stage, I use the following:

- Polyporus Combination (*Zhu Ling Tang*)
- Gentiana Combination (*Long Dan Xie Gan Tang*)
- For the chronic phase or for weaker or elderly patients I use:
- Lotus Seed Combination (*Qing Xin Lian Zi Yin*)
- Rehmannia 8 (*Ba Wei Di Huang Wan*)

Interstitial Cystitis/Painful Bladder Syndrome (IC/PBS)

One of the challenges in treating PBS, which used to be called IC, is teasing out the actual symptoms of the syndrome and figuring out what the root cause is from a Chinese medicine perspective. Is there an emotional, digestive, musculoskeletal or immune component? There is always a pain component which is usually caused by inflammation of the lining of the bladder.

Two classic formulas may be tried:

- Rehmannia 8 (*Ba Wei Di Huang Wan*)
- Lotus Seed Combination (*Qing Xin Lian Zi Yin*)

There are also a few modern formulas which have been proven to be very effective:

- Dianthus Formula (*Ba Zheng San*)
- Pyrrosia 14 (Seven Forests)
- CystiQuell (Blue Poppy Herbs)
- Intercys: Cystitis Herbal Capsules (from Dr. Qingyao Shi, OM, LAc)

Kidney Stones

In Chinese Medicine, kidney stones include stones from the kidneys and ureters as well as the urinary bladder and urethra. During the acute phase, the following two formulas can be used as a kind of "emergen-C" care to help with acute pain and discomfort:

- Rhubarb and Aconite Combination (*Dan Huang Fu Zi Tang*)
- Peony and Licorice Combination (*Shao Yao Gan Cao Tang*)

Also during the acute phase one should check for *Oketsu* and use the following formulas if the blood stasis points are palpable and elicit a pain response:

- Cinnamon and Hoelen Combination with Coix (single herb) added (*Gui Zhi Fu Ling Tang with Yi Yi Ren*)

- Rhubarb and Moutan Combination (*Dan Huang Mu Dan Pi Tang*)
- Persica and Rhubarb Combination (*Tao He Chen Qi Tang*)

At the beginning of the acute phase, if there is gas and bloating, consider using Major Zanthoxylum Combination (*Da Jian Zhong Tang*).

During the time when the stone(s) is being expelled, and there may be blood in the urine and retention of urine, use Polyporus Combination (*Zhu Ling Tang*).

Lastly, for the robust, large-sized individual who complains of fullness in the abdomen and constipation, consider using Siler and Platycodon Combination (*Fang Feng Tong Shen San*).

Conclusion

Chinese medicine and *Kanpo*, in particular, have much to offer in the area of pelvic pain and urological conditions. In conjunction with other key modalities, such as physical therapy and allopathic interventions, Chinese herbs can help many patients to improve and resolve many of these conditions. While more research needs to be done, Chinese herbs have thousands of years of empirical efficacy and offer the patient a gentler path toward a healthier state of being.

Acknowledgment

Preparation of *Kanpo* herbal medicine is taught in the old fashioned way: it is passed down by a master to an apprentice. I would like to acknowledge my mentor–teacher in these studies: Nigel Dawes, LAc, of Soho Health Arts and his post-graduate internship on *Kanpo* medicine. Many of the ideas here were gleaned from his lecture series "A Post-graduate Program in Sino-Japanese Herbal Medicine" and reflect his vast knowledge and experience in the area of Chinese herbal medicine.

References

1. Rister R. *Japanese Herbal Medicine: The Healing art of Kampo.* Avery Publishing Group; 1999.
2. Kuwaki T. *Chinese herbal therapy: A guide to its principles & practice =* [*Han fang chen liao shou ts`e*]. Long Beach, CA: Oriental Healing Arts Institute; 1990.

Chapter 3

Western Herbal Medicine

Eric Yarnell

Associate Professor, Bastyr University, Seattle, Washington

Western herbal medicines offer useful and effective treatment options for a number of benign urologic conditions. Western herbs for urinary tract infections (UTIs), overactive bladder (OAB), stress incontinence, pelvic pain syndromes in men and women, benign prostatic hyperplasia, sexual dysfunction, Peyronie's disease, phimosis, low testosterone, and kidney stones are discussed. The use of many of these herbs is based on clinical trial results, and others on historical and clinical experience. The safety and proper dosing of all agents mentioned are provided.

Introduction

The most common herbs used in North America for treating urological conditions will be considered here and are based on a combination of the author's 20 years of clinical experience and the scientific literature. Many of these herbs are of European or North American origin, but more herbs of Asian, African, South American, and Australian origin are also starting to enter the western materia medica. This chapter should not be taken as complete but as an introduction to a rich and complex subject.

Urinary Tract Infection

Western herbal medicines for lower UTI can be broken into two broad categories: those for acute treatment and those for prevention (though some agents are useful for both). These can be further subdivided into many therapeutic categories (see Table 1). While many of these herbs have a place in the treatment of complicated UTI as well, the discussion here will be limited to uncomplicated UTI.

In acute uncomplicated UTI, the most broadly applicable and effective single herb is *Juniperus* spp. (juniper) female cone (frequently but erroneously called the "berry").[1] It is most appropriate because it has three of the most important actions for

Table 1.   Summary of Western Herbal Interventions for UTI

Therapeutic Category	Treatment, Prevention or Both	Specific Agents
Urinary antiseptic	Treatment	*Juniperus* spp., *Arctostaphylos* spp., *Arbutus menziesii, Agathosma betulina, Santalum spicata, Rosmarinus officinalis*
Diuretic	Both	*Juniperus* spp., *Solidago* spp., *Urtica dioica* leaf, *Taraxacum officinale* leaf
Anti-adhesive (gut and urinary tract)	Both	*Vaccinium* spp., *Mahonia aquifolium, Hydrastis canadensis, Coptis* spp., *Berberis* spp.
Immune stimulant	Both	*Echinacea angustifolia* root
Demulcent	Treatment	*Elymus repens, Zea mays, Althaea officinalis*
Inflammation modulator	Treatment	*Eryngium yuccifolium, Solidago* spp., *Juniperus* spp.
Antibiotic resistance inhibitors	Treatment (adjunct)	*Camellia sinensis, Rosmarinus officinalis, Silybum marianum*

resolving acute UTIs: potent urinary antiseptic, potent diuretic, and moderately inflammation modulating. Many species in the genus are interchangeable as medicine, including *J. communis* (common juniper), *J. osteosperma* (Utah juniper), and *J. monosperma* (one-seed juniper).

Shockingly, given its potency and broad activity, no clinical trials could be identified on the use of juniper in patients with UTI. Animal studies have shown no toxicity for large dos es of the highly-concentrated volatile oil of juniper, or its important isolated constituent terpinen-4-ol. One study even showed juniper oil to be nephroprotective in rats exposed to tacrolimus.[2] It should be avoided in pregnancy and lactation until its safety can be assessed in these settings.

The usual dose of tincture (60% ethanol, 1:3–1:5 weight:volume (w:v) ratio) is 1–2 mL every 2–4 hours for the first 2–3 days of the UTI then three times daily until symptoms are completely resolved.

The other most common acute urinary antiseptic herbs are those containing arbutin (a glucoside containing hydroquinone, the actual antimicrobial compound), principally leaves of *Arctostaphylos uva ursi* (uva ursa) but also numerous Southwestern American/Northern Mexican species such as *A. pungens* (pointleaf manzanita) and the Pacific Northwestern species *Arbutus menziesii* (madrone). Surprisingly, as almost all sources recommend restricting use of these herbs to short-term use, the only clinical study on *uva ursi* was a double-blind trial that randomized 57 women with recurrent UTIs to either a standardized extract of *uva ursi* or placebo for one year.[3] There was a significant reduction in UTI recurrence with *uva ursi* compared to the placebo group, with no serious adverse effects.

The concern about harm from arbutin-containing herbs appears to come from extrapolation of industrial exposure to synthetic, pure hydroquinone. However, humans mostly excrete hydroquinone as glucuronides and sulfates after consumption of *uva ursi* leaves, and toxicity is almost never encountered.

The usual dose of tincture (30% ethanol, 1:3 w:v ratio) is 3–5 mL every 2–4 hours for 2–3 days then three times a day until all symptoms are gone. This may cause some digestive upset unless taken with food due to the presence of high levels of tannins. Alternatively, a cold infusion can be made from 10 g (0.33 oz) of dried leaf and as much water as desired left to soak overnight, then strained and drunk. At least three 10 g doses should be drunk each day.

Though it is frequently stated that alkaline urine is necessary for deconjugation and thus activity of arbutin from *uva ursi* and its relatives, it has been shown that uropathogens deconjugate it and thus alkaline urine is not essential. This in part explains the clinical observation that cranberry does not interfere with *uva ursi*; it is also because cranberry only very transiently and in large doses acidifies the urine of some people.[4]

Agathosma betulina (buchu) leaf, native to South Africa, and *Santalum spicata* (Australian sandalwood) volatile oil are two other useful urinary antiseptics for patients with uncomplicated acute UTIs based on clinical experience (clinical trials have not been conducted).[5] Diosphenol is an important active terpenoid in buchu. *S. album* (white sandalwood) is more commonly known than the Australian species, but its habitat is threatened and it is subject to widespread illegal harvest, resulting in it being considered vulnerable to extinction by the International Union for the Conservation of Nature. Australian sandalwood is a very similar, widely cultivated, sustainable alternative.

Buchu is significantly less potent than juniper or arbutin-containing herbs, and should generally be paired with one of them for best efficacy. The usual dose of tincture (60% ethanol, 1:4–1:5 w:v ratio) is 3–5 mL every 2–4 hours for the first 2–3 days then three times a day until symptoms completely resolve. Australian sandalwood volatile oil is extremely potent and should be kept out of reach of children. Its usual dose in adults is 3–5 drops every 3–4 hours for the first two days then three times a day until symptoms resolve. Neither should be used in pregnancy until more information is available on their safety.

Multiple aquaretic herbs are used clinically to help flush out infecting microbes, an approach confirmed as effective by the

German governmental body that assessed efficacy of herbs known as the Commission E. *Solidago canadensis* (goldenrod) flowering top, *Urtica dioica* (nettle) leaf, and *Taraxacum officinale* (dandelion) leaf are some of the most common and best-confirmed herbal aquaretics. There is some evidence that goldenrod is also antimicrobial. They are best utilized as infusions as this adds additional water, itself beneficial in UTI patients. Typical doses are one tablespoon of herb per cup of hot water steeped for at least 15 minutes. Patients should drink four or more cups per day. Ginger or other pungent flavors work best to cover the taste of these herbs without adverse effects, compared to adding sweeteners. Aquaretic herbs are very safe, including with long-term use, and can also be used for UTI prevention.

Vaccinium macrocarpon (cranberry) fruit and related species, including *V. corymbosum* (blueberry) and related species and *V. parvifolium* (evergreen huckleberry), contain type A proanthocyanidins that have repeatedly been shown to have an anti-adhesive effect against *E. coli.*[6] This makes them primarily helpful for prevention of UTIs, particularly in patients with asymptomatic bacteriuria, though they have some limited benefit as part of a treatment program for patients with acute UTIs.There are many dose forms available and they seem effective, though many patients who self-treat under dose. Capsules or tablets should provide at least 1,000 mg three times per day, and at least 8 oz. of pure cranberry juice needs to be taken daily for optimal results. Despite some case studies suggesting cranberry can cause problems combined with warfarin, multiple controlled trials have failed to show any interaction between the two.[7]

Numerous other categories of western herbs are used to treat and prevent UTI, though they have not been rigorously assessed for these purposes. *Echinacea angustifolia* (purple coneflower) root is a widely used immune stimulant, eclipsed by research on its immunomodulating cousin *E. purpurea* flowering tops due to a historical accident. Clinically purple coneflower is preferred and is mainly utilized in treating and preventing infections in patients who are known to be immunocompromised or in whom other approaches simply haven't worked. Purple coneflower should be avoided in patients with significant autoimmune diseases or those taking immunosuppressive drugs. Usual dose of tincture (70% ethanol 1:2–1:3) is 3–5 mL every 2 hours during acute infections and two to three times per day for prevention.

Numerous types of inflammation-modulating herbs are also recommended to relieve pain and irritation in patients suffering acute UTIs. *Eryngium yuccifolium* (rattlesnake master) root and demulcent herbs including *Elymus repens* (couch grass) rhizome, *Zea mays* (corn) stigmata ("silk"), and *Althaea officinalis* (marsh-mallow) root or leaf, are particularly useful in this setting based on historical and clinical use. Goldenrod and juniper are also inflammation modulating, further enhancing their utility in treating patients with UTIs. The usual dose of rattlesnake master tincture (70–80% ethanol, 1:2–1:3) is 1–3 mL every 2 hours. The usual preparation of the demulcents is as a cold infusion. Three table-spoons (roughly 15 g) chopped or powdered herb is added to 1 quarter (1 L) of water and left to sit in a warm place for 12 hours. This is strained then drunk throughout the day.

In some situations, antibiotics have to be used to treat and prevent UTIs effectively. Western herbs still have a role in such situations, as they can potentiate antibiotics and reduce resistance to them. For example, corilagin, a polyphenol found in *uva ursi* leaf, was synergistic with β-lactam antibiotics against methicillin-resistant *Staphylococcus aureus* (MRSA).[8] *Rosmarinus officinalis* (rosemary) and *Silybum marianum* (milk thistle) have also shown potential to reduce antibiotic resistance. *Camellia sinensis* (green tea) flavonoids known as catechins are believed to reduce resistance by blocking efflux pumps in microbes. There is some clinical confirmation of this from two clinical trials in elderly Japanese patients with MRSA pneumonia not responding to antibiotics who were treated with aerosolized green tea catechins.[9] Patients improved dramatically with the combination of antibiotics and green tea. However, these trials did not have control groups that compared no antibiotics and green tea alone to the combination, so it is possible that the clinical benefit was not due to reducing antibiotic resistance. Future trials should specifically investigate the exact role of western herbs in reducing antibiotic resistance. In the meantime, consider giving patients with multidrug resistant pathogens causing UTIs green tea capsules 1–2 g three times per day or one cup of tea three times per day to see if antibiotic activity can be potentiated.

Overactive Bladder/Urge Incontinence

Very little research has been done on the potential benefits of herbal spasmolytics in patients with OABs. One of the most traditional western herbs for this condition is *Hyoscyamus niger* (henbane) herb. This is a potent antimuscarinic agent that works along the same lines as drugs such as oxybutynin and tolterodine. The usual dose of tincture (50% ethanol, 1:3–1:5) is 3–5 drops three times per day. Ideally, the dose is titrated to the point that it starts to cause mild dry mouth or symptoms are relieved. In overdose, it can cause blurred vision, warm flushed skin, tachycardia, arrhythmia, agitation, confusion, urinary retention, distension of the bladder, drowsiness, hyperreflexia, aggressiveness, convulsion, delirium, hallucinations, coma, and death. Elderly patients are more susceptible to these effects and so the start dose should be low and slowly increased (by one drop per dose every day or two). It should be avoided in benign prostatic hyperplasia.

Bryophyllum pinnatum (air plant) is a succulent native to Madagascar used in traditional medicine as a spasmolytic. A randomized trial found that two capsules of the crude herb three times a day showed a trend toward superiority of placebo for reducing urinary frequency in 20 patients with OABs.[10] The herb was completely safe, which is important, as it has been reported to contain cardiac glycosides.

Other herb spasmolytics may help in this condition, but they have not been studied. These include *Viburnum prunifolium* (black haw) bark, *Dioscorea villosa* (wild yam) rhizome, and others that will be discussed in the section under kidney stones.

Stress Incontinence

There is also very little information about what western herbs are effective for stress incontinence. *Ephedra sinica* (ma huang) stem and its alkaloid ephedrine, which is a mixed alpha- and beta-adrenergic agonist (the former increases urethral resistance), is the best understood natural agent for stress incontinence. In an open study of elderly patients with stress incontinence, oral ephedrine improved symptoms without objectively changing cystometric findings. In a series of women with chronic stress incontinence after hysterectomy, oral ephedrine was very effective, though it quickly lost efficacy in women with total sphincter failure.[11] Twelve of 16 schizophrenic patients who had incontinence due to clozapine (which is, in part, an alpha antagonist) had this complication completed resolved (and all improved) on ephedrine up to 150 mg per day.[12]

The lowest observed adverse effect level for ephedrine is 150 mg; this dose should not be exceeded. At typical doses of tincture (50% ethanol, 1:3 w:v, 5–30 drops three times per day), at most 15–30 mg of ephedrine are delivered. However, the tincture contains multiple alkaloids and other constituents that may act synergistically. In overdose, it can cause hypertension, anxiety, restlessness, tachycardia, and insomnia. It is contraindicated in patients with hypertension or pre-existing anxiety disorders.

In mice, cinnamaldehyde from *Cinnamomum* spp. (cinnamon) bark reduced stress incontinence without causing hypertension.[13] Its mechanism of action remains to be determined, but it appeared to involve inducible nitric oxide synthase and superoxide dismutase.

IC/PBS/Pelvic Pain/Chronic Prostatitis

Many categories of herbs are used to treat pelvic pain in men and women, mostly empirically. Demulcents (which may also act as urothelial restoratives), bladder analgesics, bladder tonics, and skeletal muscle relaxants, along with inflammation modulators, are the most important of these. Various herbs are usually used in combination, as opposed to singly.

Piper methysticum (kava) root and *Pedicularis* spp. (lousewort) flowering top are clinically the most effective pelvic analgesics. Kava's role in treating pelvic pain has been somewhat forgotten in the past 100 years, but at least since the late 1800s, the Eclectics (medical doctors in North America who basically practiced naturopathic medicine) recognized kava as a specific treatment for pelvic pain. It has been studied as an analgesic and a meta-analysis of clinical trials confirms it is a systemic anxiolytic.[14] It is therefore most indicated in pelvic pain patients who have concomitant anxiety, which is quite common. Lousewort has not received any research attention but empirically works just like kava, if not better, and actually tastes good. Both kava and lousewort are also effective skeletal muscle relaxants and are empirically useful in the subset of pelvic pain patients who have pelvic floor dysfunction at the root of their problems.

Kava can be taken as a capsule or tincture. The usual adult dose is 500–1,000 mg of crude root 2–3 times per day in capsules or a 70% ethanol tincture, 1:2–1:3 w:v, 1–3 mL 2–3 times per day. The dose of lousewort tincture is the same, but it is made at just 30–50% ethanol (it is not available in capsules).

Kava has an undeserved reputation for hepatotoxicity that was based on a gross exaggeration of a handful of cases. Given the millions of users every day, the rate of harm is extremely low and fits best with a pattern of idiosyncratic reaction rather than consistent hepatotoxicity of the herb. For greatest safety, it should be avoided in patients with severe liver diseases, but otherwise serum transaminases do not need to be monitored or any other precautions taken. Leaf and stem extracts should not be used, as it is unclear if they were responsible for some of the cases of toxicity. Lousewort is generally very safe, though it depends where it was harvested, as it is hemiparasitic and could uptake harmful constituents from toxic plants if growing very near them.

Cornsilk, couch grass, and marshmallow were previously mentioned as inflammation-modulating demulcents in the setting of UTI. They are also widely used clinically in patients with IC and chronic prostatitis and are often reported to reduce pain. Though frequently said to be diuretic, one human trial did not confirm this for cornsilk.[15] This is a positive, as many patients with chronic pelvic pain (CPP) syndromes already have urinary frequency so diuretics are often contraindicated. Instead, it is believed that demulcents decrease inflammation and possibly repair urothelial leakage, but no research has been done on this question. Dosing these herbs is discussed under UTI above.

Secale cereale (rye) pollen is an inflammation modulator and has been studied in several randomized, double-blind trials in men with chronic abacterial prostatitis and CPP syndrome. At least two trials (one three months, one six months) found it superior to placebo for reducing symptoms monitored using the standard NIH-CPSI questionnaire.[16] One double-blind trial found it enhanced the efficacy of levofloxacin compared to rye pollen and placebo.[17] The usual dose of an aqueous/acetone extract (63 mg/cap) is 2 caps bid–tid. It should be avoided in people with celiac disease. It is otherwise very safe.

Quercetin is a flavonoid found in most plants. One double blind, randomized trial compared quercetin 500 mg tid to placebo reduced symptoms in men with chronic abacterial prostatitis.[18] It is believed to work as an inflammation modulator and is extremely safe.

Benign Prostatic Hyperplasia (BPH)

Western herbs for BPH fall into two broad categories: those treating underlying mechanisms and those that treat symptoms. Some herbs do both, such as *Serenoa repens* (saw palmetto) fruit, one of the best researched of all western herbs. There is some evidence of its traditional use as a prostate tonic, but it only became widely known after extensive clinical research began on highly-refined extracts in Germany in the 1950s. This native of the southeastern US and the Caribbean is almost entirely harvested from the wild in Florida.

The research on saw palmetto neatly illustrates a common theme in western herbal medicine: multiple constituents act on multiple pathways mildly, adding up to a clinically relevant effect, at least in some patients.[19] Among the many actions saw palmetto's fatty acids and phytosterols have include non-specific 5α-reductase inhibition, phytoestrogen, α1 adrenergic antagonist, inducing apoptosis in hyperplastic cells, calcium channel blockers, and epidermal growth factor receptor antagonist.[19] Compared to finasteride, saw palmetto extracts inhibit types 1 and 2 5α-reductase by 32–50% compared to 80% for type 2 only with the drug. This results in an absence of adverse effects with saw palmetto extract seen with finasteride such as low libido and sexual dysfunction, but also means that saw palmetto does not appreciably shrink the prostate.

The most recent meta-analysis of clinical trials of saw palmetto extracts contains a contradiction that is hard to reconcile.[20] According to this study, saw palmetto extracts are not superior to placebo at lowering overall BPH-related symptoms (based on the International Prostate Symptom Score (IPSS), the standard instrument used in clinical trials), improving peak flower, or reducing nocturia. The same meta-analysis concluded that saw palmetto extracts are just as effective as tamsulosin. The largest (n = 1,098) single randomized double-blind trial of saw palmetto extract found it was just as effective as finasteride for men with prostates under 50 cc with mild-to-moderate symptoms.[21] Saw palmetto resulted in far fewer adverse effects than finasteride in this head-to-head comparison trial. It is not logical that saw palmetto is simultaneously as effective as conventional drugs for BPH and not superior to placebo. Either conventional drugs are also not superior to placebo, or else there is some problem with the trial design in the saw palmetto vs. placebo trials.

Given the low cost of this agent, ease of use, its extreme good safety record, long-term (two year) open trials saying it can reduce the risk of progression and need for surgery, and the fact that it clearly does help some patients clinically, it is worth considering saw palmetto extracts to prevent and treat men with BPH. The usual dose of standardized extracts containing 70–90% fatty acids and sterols is 320 mg once per day.

Prunus africanum (pygeum) bark is frequently discussed as another herbal remedy for BPH with a similar chemical profile, set of actions, and safety as saw palmetto. It is, however, not recommended for use in North America for ecological reasons. Unlikely saw palmetto's fruit, which is harvested without harming the plant, taking the bark from pygeum easily kills the trees. Also, because it grows primarily in impoverished areas in Africa, there is perverse incentive for desperately poor people to unsustainably harvest the bark of the tree to get as much money as possible. Unfortunately, the trees do not grow in thick stands but are scattered and uncommon, and most of the profit from pygeum goes to primarily European supplements manufacturers who create extracts and not local African people. While there is some hope that locally-managed, sustainable, cultivated stands will become more common and that more profits will go to local people, this is far from the reality. There is simply no reason at present to ship this product across the ocean when a sustainable, well-characterized, cheap, effective alternative exists much closer by. Patients and practitioners in Europe and Africa are encouraged to use only products sourced from sustainable cooperative growers.

Urtica dioica (nettle) root, quite distinctly from its diuretic leaf, is a sex hormone-binding globulin (SHBG) receptor and synthesis inhibitor, as well as an aromatase inhibitor, due to a range of constituents. Large controlled trials continue to show it is effective for relieving symptoms in men with mild-to-moderate BPH.[22] A combination of nettle root and saw palmetto has been shown superior to finasteride at relieving BPH symptoms, with far fewer adverse effects.[23] This safe herb should be used routinely for at least six months to determine if it will be helpful. The usual dose of crude herb extracts is 500–1,000 mg bid–tid.

Table 2. Miscellaneous Herbs for BPH

Herb	Dose	Notes on Use
Cucurbita pepo (pumpkin) seed oil	1,000 mg tid	Slow to take effect (use six month minimum)
Ganoderma lucidum (reishi, ling zhi) mycelium and fruiting body	1,000–3,000 mg tid	Also an ACE inhibitor and adaptogenic/ immunomodulating
Secale cereale (rye) pollen	Aqueous/acetone extract (63 mg/cap) 2 bid–tid	Likely interferes with growth factors (use six month minimum)
Ammi visnaga (khella) fruit	Tincture (50% etoh, 1:3 w:v) 1–2 mL tid	Rapid-onset spasmolytic
Epilobium spp. (small-flowered willow herb) flowering top	Tincture (30% etoh, 1:3 w:v) 3–5 mL tid	Slow to take effect (use six month minimum)

Note: All of these herbs are recommended for use in combination with other herbs and not as single therapeutic agents

Quite a few other herbs have been studied for their effects on men with BPH, though their mechanisms of action are poorly understood. Others have been found useful clinically but haven't yet been the subject of formal clinical trials. These herbs are summarized in Table 2.

One approach to using western herbs for men with BPH is to start with strong spasmolytics such as khella for two weeks, particularly in men with smaller (<50 cc) prostates. If this works, it both confirms that they have spasmodic BPH and that the herb is effective. Saw palmetto and nettle root can then be added to prevent worsening of the disease and growth of the prostate over time. If khella doesn't work, then a combination of a range of the other herbs mentioned should be implemented for at least six months. If there is no improvement, and the prostate is >50 cc, then finasteride or dutasteride should be used (or surgery in extreme cases) to get the prostate back below 50 cc, and then at least saw palmetto and nettle root (along with lifestyle changes) implemented to prevent recurrence.

Sexual Dysfunction

Erectile dysfunction (ED) is a symptom of some other underlying dysfunction that must be identified and treated, particularly arteriosclerosis and diabetes.[24] *Allium sativum* (garlic) bulb may be the ultimate treatment for ED due to arteriosclerosis, given that it both has direct benefits on sexual function in men as well as having been shown to actually reverse arteriosclerotic plaques.[25] While treating causes is underway, symptomatic relief is desirable. Western herbal medicine offers the potential to help diagnose the cause of the ED, treat the underlying problem(s), and bring symptomatic relief. Major treatments are discussed in the text; see Table 3 for less well-established herbs. It should be noted that combination products sold over the counter are extremely likely to

Table 3.   Miscellaneous Herbs for ED

Herb and Part Used	Possible Mechanism(s)	Dose
Crocus sativus (saffron) stigmata	Central-acting aphrodisiac	15–30 mg bid
Butea superba (red kwao krua) tuber	Unknown (if any)	Unknown/not recommended
Epimedium spp. (horny goat weed, *yin yang* huo) leaf	Its flavonoid icariin is PDE5i and enhances eNOS expression	Granulation 3 g tid; tincture 1–2 mL tid
Eurycoma longifolia (tomcat ali) root and bark	Possible aromatase inhibitor	300 mg aqueous extract qd. Use caution, frequently adulterated with PDE5i drugs
Lepidium meyenii (maca) tuber	Unknown (possibly as a non-specific adaptogen)	3–10 g powder qd
Tribulus terrestris (caltrop vine) herb	Endothelium/nitric oxide-related penile vasodilator	Tincture 1–2 mL tid

Abbreviations: eNOS = endothelial nitric oxide synthase; PDE5i = phosphodiesterase type 5 inhibitor; SSRI = selective serotonin reuptake inhibitor be adulterated with PDE-5 inhibitor drugs and only brands of well-established herbs from respected companies should be used.[26]

Pausinystalia yohimbe (yohimbe) bark contains alkaloids, notably yohimbine, that are central, presynaptic, α2-adrenergic receptor antagonists, functionally acting like norepinephrine reuptake inhibitors.[27] Yohimbe is thus primarily a libido enhancer and antidepressant. Meta-analysis of clinical trials confirms that pure yohimbine is effective for men with ED with only minor adverse effects.[28] Yohimbine is not currently available as a prescription drug, only yohimbe and various combination supplements containing pure yohimbine of dubious safety (though even in these cases, most adverse effects are mild and associated with inappropriate use by lay people). However, it is most likely to work in depressed men with low libido. It has also been shown to be effective in offsetting low libido caused by SSRI antidepressant medications in women as well as men.[29]

Clinically, yohimbe can be used as one way to try to determine the extent of psychological vs. physical ED. If after two weeks of therapy with yohimbe there is substantial improvement in ED, then almost certainly the problem is primarily psychogenic. If there is minimal improvement, there is a greater chance of a more serious underlying physical problem (most likely, metabolic syndrome, diabetes, or arteriosclerosis).

The usual therapeutic dose of a 1:3 tincture of yohimbe (50% ethanol) is 3–5 drops twice per day. The therapeutic dose of pure yohimbine is 5.4 mg qd–bid. Combining yohimbe with argining 6 g per day may augment its efficacy. There is evidence from animal studies that yohimbine and sildenafil work well together and may offset each other's opposite but negative effects on blood pressure.[30] Yohimbe is contraindicated in men with hypertension and anxiety disorders including post-traumatic stress. Blood pressure has to be monitored regularly in men taking yohimbe and the herb discontinued if blood pressure goes up.

Milder aphrodisiacs (herbs that increase libido) can also be used in cases of men with psychogenic ED. *Turnera diffusa* (damiana) flowering top is one of the best known with a long tradition of use for this purpose. Though human trials are lacking, animal studies confirm it increases libido. It may also have vasodilating properties and thus also work peripherally.[31] Clinically, its effects are mild so long-term use (several months) is recommended. Typical doses of tincture (60% ethanol, 1:3–1:4 w:v) are 2–3 mL tid. It is safe for use in women as well.

Panax ginseng (Asian ginseng) root (particularly red ginseng, which is the steamed then dried root of four-year-old Asian ginseng plants) and fruit have been extensively studied for its effects on men with ED. Trials starting in the early 1990s confirm that red ginseng is superior to placebo and trazodone for improving erection quality and duration as well as libido. A meta-analysis of clinical trials confirmed that Asian ginseng is effective for treating men with ED.[32] The fruit of Asian ginseng has also proven effective compared to placebo in double-blind trials, again improving both erectile quality and sexual desire.[33] The usual dose of red ginseng powder is 3–5 g bid. A combination of standardized extract of red ginseng with *Ginkgo biloba* leaf extract, arginine, and various minerals and vitamins has been shown effective in clinical trials in men and women with sexual dysfunction.[34] It generally has no adverse effects but if it causes insomnia should only be taken in the morning. Note that wild Asian ginseng is critically endangered and only cultivated material should ever be used, and is generally all that is available.

Peyronie's Disease

Peyronie's disease is a fibrotic condition affecting the tunica albuginea of the penis. It can lead to acute and chronic penile curvature, pain and/or ED. *Centella astiatica* (gotu kola) whole plant is a very safe antifibrotic herb, notably inhibiting transforming growth factor 1β which is overexpressed in Peyronie's disease plaques.[35] Gotu extracts are helpful in conditions such as systemic sclerosis which involve pathogenic mechanisms similar to Peyronie's disease.[36] Clinically, applying a cream that is 50% gotu kola tincture or glycerite by volume twice daily for up to six month has been very helpful in reducing pain and inflammation while improving erectile function. It so far has not reduced palpable plaques or penile curvature.

Phimosis

There is no research on herbal treatments for phimosis. Gotu kola applied in a manner very similar to that described under Peyronie's disease has also proven clinically helpful. Research is urgently needed to determine if this is a viable alternative to topical corticosteroids.

Low Testosterone

No herbal medicine has been shown to increase testosterone synthesis or secretion in controlled clinical trials (see Table 4). Open trials suggesting testosterone elevations have been of poor quality and not confirmed in the more rigorous, randomized follow-up trails cited in Table 4.[37] Many herbs purported to be testosterone boosters were traditionally used as tonics in older men, but obviously traditional people had no knowledge of testosterone, and there is no clear correlation between the symptoms of aging and levels of testosterone in men except at the more extreme ends of the population anyway. Thus, while tonic herbs for older men may have clinical value, it is unlikely to be through androgen elevation.

Table 4. Negative Clinical Trials on Reputed Testosterone-Enhancing Herbs

Herb	Part Used
Eurycoma longifolia (tongkat ali)	Root and bark
Lepidium meyenii (maca)	Tuber
Tribulus terrestris (caltrop vine)	Flower top in fruit

Kidney Stones

Herbs related to kidney stones can be grouped into two major groups: those that help with acute stone passage and those that help prevent stones. One category of herb crosses over between these categories: diuretics. Some of the more potent and commonly used western herbal diuretics (several of which have already been discussed earlier in this chapter) include juniper, nettle leaf, dandelion leaf, goldenrod, *Apium graveolens* (celery) fruit or root, *Levisticum officinale* (lovage) leaf, *Petroselinum crispum* (parsley) root, *Taraxacum officinale* (dandelion) leaf, and *Equisetum* spp. (horsetail) herb. When coupled with strong spasmolytic herbs to control the pain of ureteral colic, diuretic herbs can continue to push the stones out.

Unfortunately, this approach has mostly only been validated in clinical practice using the herbs mentioned. However, there is full evidence from multiple randomized trials that a combination of the herbal terpenoids pinene, camphene, borneol, anethole, fenchone, and cineol dissolved in olive oil results in better stone passage rates than placebo and equal rates compared to alpha blocker drugs.[38] While this may be primarily due to the spasmolytic nature of these terpenoids, this does give at least some support to the idea that herbs could be useful in patients with acute ureteral colic.

Ammi visnaga (khella) fruit is one of the more effective ureteral spasmolytics in practice. At a dose of just 1–2 mL of tincture (1:2–1:3 w:v ratio, 30–40% ethanol) 3–5 times per day, it can effectively suppress pain due to stone passage. At least one published case study supports this observation. In preclinical models, this herb has also been shown to protect renal epithelium from damage by oxalate crystals and to prevent calcium oxalate crystal deposition in the kidneys.[39] This herb is very safe at these doses and is an excellent first-line spasmolytic in acute stone patients. *Piscidia piscipula* (Jamaican dogwood) bark is effective at similar doses, but is much rarer and more threatened, so should be considered a second-line therapy. *Lobelia inflata* (lobelia) flowering top in fruit is actually more potent than khella but easily causes significant digestive upset, so should be used with caution in these patients who are often already nauseated. Doses of lobelia tincture or acetract (1:3–1:5 w:v, 50% ethanol) are 10 drops 3–5 times per day initially (increase by one drop per dose to gut tolerance).

Many other herbs can reduce the risk of stone formation in the first place, and some may also help dissolve very slowly stones in the kidney that are not passing.[40] The latter are typically known as litholytics. All diuretic herbs may fit both categories as either increase urinary volume and may also improve various urine parameters important to preventing stone crystallization. Several of the herbs used for these purposes and that have at least preliminary validation in human clinical trials are discussed below. See Table 5 for a listing of other potential litholytics.

Phyllanthus niuri (chanca piedra) herb is a traditional litholytic; its Spanish common name translates as "stone breaker." In a randomized trial, 69 patients with a history of calcium stone formation took either Chanca piedra powder 450 mg tid or placebo for

Table 5. Miscellaneous Potential Litholytic Herbs

Herb	Part Used	Research Notes
Hibiscus sabdariffa (roselle)	Flower	Infusion uricosuric in stone formers
Tribulus terrestris (caltrop vine)	Herb in fruit	Prevents kidney stones in rats. Prevents hyperoxaluria due to sodium glycolate feeding in rats
Herniaria hirsuta (restharrow)	Herb	Prevents calcium oxalate stones in rats
Eupatorium purpureum (Joe Pye weed)	Root	Traditional litholytic; no research located on its efficacy. Avoid in patients with renal or liver failure due to possible presence of unsaturated pyrrolizidine alkaloids
Rubia tinctorium, R. cordifolia (madder)	Root	Prevents kidney stones due to ethylene glycol in rats
Orthosiphon stamineus (Java tea)	Leaf, flower	Traditionally used as diuretic, but failed to decrease calcium stone formation in rats

three months.[41] Among patients with baseline hypercalciuria, there was a significant reduction in urinary calcium in the chanca piedra group compared to controls. In a randomized trial, 150 patients undergoing extracorporeal shockwave lithotripsy for calcium oxalate stones took either a chanca piedra extract 2 g daily or no treatment for three months.[42] Lower caliceal stone-free rates were significantly higher in the chanca piedra group, though retreatment rates were not different between the groups. Chanca piedra is very safe and it appears that it could, if the optimal form and dose could be determined, play a role in preventing kidney stones.

A proprietary tincture formula containing three herbs, *Centaurium erythraea* (common centaury) leaf, lovage root, and *Rosmarinus officinalis* (rosemary) leaf, at a dose of 50 gtt tid has been shown in open trials lasting up to four months to increase urinary output and magnesium levels while lowering calcium and oxalate levels significantly compared to baseline in idiopathic calcium stone formers.

Taking 3 oz of *Aloe vera* (aloe) gel twice per day lowered urine oxalate excretion in healthy adult males in an open trial.[43] Infusions of *Achillea fillipendulina* (fernleaf yarrow) flowering top and *Mentha* x *piperita* (peppermint) leaf were diuretic and decreased calcium oxalate crystallization in calcium stone patients.[44]

Macrotyloma uniflorum var *uniflorum* (horse gram, kulattha), formerly *Dolichos biflorus*, is a bean that has some history of use to prevent kidney stones. In a six month, randomized trial, horse gram powder was compared to potassium citrate in 47 patients with calcium-containing kidney stones.[45] Stone size shrank significantly (mean 1.2 mm) in the horse gram but not the potassium citrate group compared to baseline.

Conclusion

Western herbal medicine has much to offer to patients with benign urological conditions of many types. Sociopolitical factors, particularly lack of financial incentives like those seen with pharmaceutical development and weakness of government-funded research programs, have limited the amount of research available to assess the efficacy of traditional herbal medicines in this field. These herbs have been in continuous use for thousands of years and continue to be widely used, and their empirical efficacy is at least part of the reason for this ongoing practice.[46] More research is warranted, and at least those best-confirmed can be implemented in practice now. It is particularly important that future studies compare herbs to drugs directly (including efficacy, safety, and cost) to get the best sense of their place in modern medicine.

Western herbal medicine is safe. This is not to say herbs are free of risk, but given their very high level of use they result in a shockingly low level of reports of toxicity, particularly compared to pharmaceutical drugs, which carry high burdens of toxicity despite proper use. The excellent safety record of western herbal medicine combined with its relatively low cost alone recommends it for further research and wider implementation.

References

1. Blumenthal M and Busse WR. *The complete German Commission E monographs.* Austin, Tex.; Boston: American Botanical Council; Integrative Medicine Communications; 1998.
2. Butani L, Afshinnik A, Johnson J, *et al.* Amelioration of tacrolimus-induced nephrotoxicity in rats using juniper oil. *Transplantation.* 2003;76(2):306–311.
3. Larsson B, Jonasson A and Fianu S. Prophylactic effect of UVA-E in women with recurrent cystitis: A preliminary report. *Curr Ther Res.* 1993;53(4):441–443.
4. Kahn HD, Panariello VA, Saeli J, Sampson JR and Schwartz E. Effect of cranberry juice on urine. *J Am Diet Assoc.* 1967;51(3):251–254.
5. Lis-Balchin M, Hart S and Simpson E. Buchu (Agathosma betulina and A. crenulata, Rutaceae) essential oils: their pharmacological action on guinea-pig ileum and antimicrobial activity on microorganisms. *J Pharm Pharmacol.* 2001;53(4):579–582.
6. Blumberg JB, Camesano TA, Cassidy A, *et al.* Cranberries and their bioactive constituents in human health. *Adv Nutr.* 2013;4(6): 618–632.

7. Zikria J, Goldman R and Ansell J. Cranberry juice and warfarin: when bad publicity trumps science. *Am J Med.* 2010;123(5):384–392.

8. Shiota S, Shimizu M, Sugiyama J, Morita Y, Mizushima T and Tsuchiya T. Mechanisms of action of corilagin and tellimagrandin I that remarkably potentiate the activity of beta-lactams against methicillin-resistant Staphylococcus aureus. *Microbiol Immunol.* 2004;48(1):67–73.

9. Yamada H, Tateishi M, Harada K, *et al.* A randomized clinical study of tea catechin inhalation effects on methicillin-resistant Staphylococcus aureus in disabled elderly patients. *J Am Med Dir Assoc.* 2006;7(2):79–83.

10. Betschart C, von Mandach U, Seifert B, *et al.* Randomized, double-blind placebo-controlled trial with Bryophyllum pinnatum versus placebo for the treatment of overactive bladder in postmenopausal women. *Phytomedicine.* 2013;20(3–4):351–358.

11. Kadar N and Nelson JH, Jr. Treatment of urinary incontinence after radical hysterectomy. *Obstet Gynecol.* 1984;64(3):400–405.

12. Fuller MA, Borovicka MC, Jaskiw GE, Simon MR, Kwon K and Konicki PE. Clozapine-induced urinary incontinence: incidence and treatment with ephedrine. *J Clin Psychiatry.* 1996;57(11):514–518.

13. Chen YH, Lin YN, Chen WC, Hsieh WT and Chen HY. Treatment of stress urinary incontinence by cinnamaldehyde, the major constituent of the chinese medicinal herb ramulus cinnamomi. *Evid Based Complement Alternat Med.* 2014;2014:280204.

14. Jamieson DD, Duffield PH. The antinociceptive actions of kava components in mice. *Clin Exp Pharmacol Physiol.* 1990;17(7):495–507.

15. Doan DD, Nguyen NH, Doan HK, *et al.* Studies on the individual and combined diuretic effects of four Vietnamese traditional herbal remedies (Zea mays, Imperata cylindrica, Plantago major and Orthosiphon stamineus). *J Ethnopharmacol.* 1992;36(3): 225–231.

16. Elist J. Effects of pollen extract preparation Prostat/Poltit on lower urinary tract symptoms in patients with chronic nonbacterial prostatitis/chronic pelvic pain syndrome: a randomized, double-blind, placebo-controlled study. *Urology.* 2006;67(1):60–63.

17. Ye ZQ, Lan RZ, Wang SG, *et al.* A clinical study of prostat combined with an antibiotic for chronic nonbacterial prostatitis. *Zhonghua Nan Ke Xue.* 2006;12(9):807–810.

18. Shoskes DA, Zeitlin SI, Shahed A and Rajfer J. Quercetin in men with category III chronic prostatitis: a preliminary prospective, double-blind, placebo-controlled trial. *Urology.* 1999;54(6):960–963.

19. Koch E. Extracts from fruits of saw palmetto (Sabal serrulata) and roots of stinging nettle (Urtica dioica): viable alternatives in the medical treatment of benign prostatic hyperplasia and associated lower urinary tracts symptoms. *Planta Med.* 2001;67(6): 489–500.

20. Tacklind J, Macdonald R, Rutks I, Stanke JU and Wilt TJ. Serenoa repens for benign prostatic hyperplasia. *Cochrane Database Syst Rev.* 2012;12:Cd001423.

21. Carraro JC, Raynaud JP, Koch G, *et al.* Comparison of phytotherapy (Permixon) with finasteride in the treatment of benign prostate hyperplasia: a randomized international study of 1,098 patients. *Prostate.* 1996;29(4):231–240; discussion 241–232.

22. Safarinejad MR. Urtica dioica for treatment of benign prostatic hyperplasia: a prospective, randomized, double-blind, placebo-controlled, crossover study. *J Herb Pharmacother.* 2005;5(4):1–11.

23. Sokeland J and Albrecht J. [Combination of Sabal and Urtica extract vs. finasteride in benign prostatic hyperplasia (Aiken stages I to II). Comparison of therapeutic effectiveness in a one year double-blind study]. *Urologe A.* 1997;36(4):327–333.

24. Miner M, Nehra A, Jackson G, *et al.* All men with vasculogenic erectile dysfunction require a cardiovascular workup. *Am J Med.* 2014; 127(3):174–182.

25. Nishimatsu H, Kitamura T, Yamada D, *et al.* Improvement of symptoms of aging in males by a preparation LEOPIN ROYAL containing aged garlic extract and other five of natural medicines — comparison with traditional herbal medicines (Kampo). *Aging Male.* 2014;17(2):112–116.

26. Gilard V, Balayssac S, Tinaugus A, Martins N, Martino R and Malet-Martino M. Detection, identification and quantification by 1H NMR of adulterants in 150 herbal dietary supplements marketed for improving sexual performance. *J Pharm Biomed Anal.* 2015;102: 476–493.

27. Goldberg MR and Robertson D. Yohimbine: a pharmacological probe for study of the alpha 2-adrenoreceptor. *Pharmacol Rev.* 1983;35(3):143–180.

28. Ernst E and Pittler MH. Yohimbine for erectile dysfunction: a systematic review and meta-analysis of randomized clinical trials. *J Urol.* 1998;159(2):433–436.

29. Michelson D, Kociban K, Tamura R and Morrison MF. Mirtazapine, yohimbine or olanzapine augmentation therapy for serotonin reuptake-associated female sexual dysfunction: a randomized, placebo controlled trial. *J Psychiatr Res.* 2002;36(3):147–152.

30. Senbel AM and Mostafa T. Yohimbine enhances the effect of sildenafil on erectile process in rats. *Int J Impot Res.* 2008;20(4):409–417.

31. Hnatyszyn O, Moscatelli V, Garcia J, *et al.* Argentinian plant extracts with relaxant effect on the smooth muscle of the corpus cavernosum of guinea pig. *Phytomedicine.* 2003;10(8):669–674.

32. Jang DJ, Lee MS, Shin BC, Lee YC and Ernst E. Red ginseng for treating erectile dysfunction: a systematic review. *Br J Clin Pharmacol.* 2008;66(4):444–450.

33. Choi YD, Park CW, Jang J, *et al.* Effects of Korean ginseng berry extract on sexual function in men with erectile dysfunction: a multicenter, placebo-controlled, double-blind clinical study. *Int J Impot Res.* 2013;25(2):45–50.

34. Ito T, Kawahara K, Das A and Strudwick W. The effects of ArginMax, a natural dietary supplement for enhancement of male sexual function. *Hawaii Med J.* 1998;57(12):741–744.

35. Bian D, Zhang J, Wu X, *et al.* Asiatic acid isolated from Centella asiatica inhibits TGF-beta1-induced collagen expression in human keloid fibroblasts via PPAR-gamma activation. *Int J Biol Sci.* 2013;9(10):1032–1042.

36. Guseva NG, Starovoitova MN and Mach ES. Madecassol treatment of systemic and localized scleroderma. *Ter Arkh.* 1998;70(5):58–61.

37. Tambi MI, Imran MK and Henkel RR. Standardised water-soluble extract of Eurycoma longifolia, Tongkat ali, as testosterone booster for managing men with late-onset hypogonadism? *Andrologia.* 2012;44 Suppl 1:226–230.

38. Chua ME, Park JH, Castillo JC and Morales ML, Jr. Terpene compound drug as medical expulsive therapy for ureterolithiasis: a meta-analysis. *Urolithiasis.* 2013;41(2):143–151.

39. Vanachayangkul P, Byer K, Khan S and Butterweck V. An aqueous extract of Ammi visnaga fruits and its constituents khellin and visnagin prevent cell damage caused by oxalate in renal epithelial cells. *Phytomedicine.* 2010;17(8–9):653–658.

40. Butterweck V and Khan SR. Herbal medicines in the management of urolithiasis: alternative or complementary? *Planta Med.* 2009;75(10): 1095–1103.
41. Nishiura JL, Campos AH, Boim MA, Heilberg IP and Schor N. Phyllanthus niruri normalizes elevated urinary calcium levels in calcium stone forming (CSF) patients. *Urol Res.* 2004;32(5):362–366.
42. Micali S, Sighinolfi MC, Celia A, *et al.* Can Phyllanthus niruri affect the efficacy of extracorporeal shock wave lithotripsy for renal stones? A randomized, prospective, long-term study. *J Urol.* 2006;176(3):1020–1022.
43. Kirdpon S, Kirdpon W, Airarat W, Trevanich A and Nanakorn S. Effect of aloe (Aloe vera Linn.) on healthy adult volunteers: changes in urinary composition. *J Med Assoc Thai.* 2006;89 Suppl 2:S9–S14.
44. Kariev SS, Gaybullaev AA and Tursunov B. E186 Phytotherapy of urolithiasis: Are extracts from medicinal plants only diuretics or are they really able to change the activity of lithogenesis? *Eur Urol Suppl.* 2015;12(3):80.
45. Singh RG, Behura SK and Kumar R. Litholytic property of Kulattha (Dolichous biflorus) vs. potassium citrate in renal calculus disease: a comparative study. *J Assoc Physicians India.* 2010;58:286–289.
46. Beck L. *De materia medica by Pedanius Dioscorides (review).* Oxford University Press; 2006.

Chapter 4

Naturopathy

Geo Espinosa and Ralph Esposito Jr

Naturopathic Doctor, Integrative Urology Specialist, Department of Urology, New York University, Langone Medical Center, New York

Naturopathy is an alternative form of medicine that employs a spectrum of natural methods that avoid the use of surgery and drugs. This approach can be helpful for people suffering from a variety of urological conditions. This chapter will explore the many avenues healthcare professionals can take in order to address these conditions. It will discuss herbal regimens and supplements along with nutritional counseling to alleviate the symptoms of different these urological illnesses.

Introduction

Naturopathy, also known as naturopathic medicine, is based on the belief that nature possesses the power to heal the patient experiencing illness. It is a system of alternative medicine where practitioners attempt to understand the origin of the sickness by understanding all elements of the person, such as their mind, body, and spirit. Because it is holistic in nature this practice relies on comprehending how all these elements work in tandem contributing to the health concern.

The two main principles of naturopathic are: empowering the individual to make lifestyle changes and supporting the individual to use their own body's healing ability. In order to achieve this, naturopaths apply different therapies such as nutritional counseling, acupuncture, detoxification, spirituality, and lifestyle counseling. These types of practices can be especially helpful when dealing with urological disorders. Naturopaths can work with the patient understanding their emotions and diet to create a health plan to alleviate symptoms or cure the body of the disorder. The following chapter will explore different approaches to address the incidences of these conditions. It will focus on dietary approaches and supplementation dosing that have been helpful to others.

Urinary Tract Infections (UTIs)

Each year approximately 8.6 million Americans visit their healthcare provider seeking treatment for UTIs which is estimated to cost $3.5 million in evaluation and treatment.[1] With the increase in pharmaceutical antibiotic resistant uropathogens,[2] the need for complementary and alternative treatments for UTIs is increasingly necessary as a first line therapy.

Dietary approach

Diet is essential in creating an environment hostile to pathogenic bacteria. Sugar may decrease immune phagocytic, neutrophil activity,[3] it is suggested patients minimize sugar, refined carbohydrate intake and dilute fruit juice. Proper hydration is essential for genitourinary (GU) health. Increasing urine flow helps flush and decrease the time pathogens may have to adhere and replicate in the GU tract. Fluid intake should be emphasized to at least 2 L/day including 0.5 L of 100% cranberry juice or 0.25 L of blueberry juice per day. Herbal tea and water are beneficial while soft drinks, coffee and alcohol may be irritating.[4] Garlic (*Allium sativum*) and onions

(*A. cepa*) should be eaten liberally and become a staple of the daily diet. The *Allium* family has a strong antimicrobial effect on common UTI pathogens such as *E. coli, Proteus* spp., *Kelbseilla pneumonia, Staphylococcus* spp., and *Streptococcus* spp.

Supplementation

D-Mannose: This simple sugar, has shown in animal and *in vitro* studies to prevent adhesion of bacterial fimbriae to uroepithelial tissue, inhibiting uropathogens growth. A human clinical randomized controlled study showed D-Mannose (2 g/day) to prophylactically prevent UTI recurrence, similarly to nitrofurantoin.[5]

- **Dosing:**
    - Prevention: 2 g (0.4 tsp) per day in water — preferably before bed
    - For acute treatment: 0.75 tsp three times per day

Botanicals

Cranberry (*Vaccinium macrocarpon*): Cranberry's long anti-UTI reputation has validity, as it prevents bacteria fimbriae type 1 (mannose specific) and P (α-D-Gal(1→4)-β-D-Gal specific) from adhering to the gut wall and urinary bladder.[6] An early study showed 73% of individuals (44 women, 15 men) consuming 0.5 L/day of cranberry juice had beneficial effects on active UTIs with cessation of cranberry resulting in recurrence.[7] Even as little as 300 mL of cranberry juice may reduce infection recurrence.[8] Some studies show equal benefit of cranberry juice vs. extract, yet other studies showed no benefit. One of the most comprehensive meta-analysis to date shows protective benefits of both cranberry juice and tablets, especially in women with recurrent UTIs and children.[9]

- **Dosing:**
    - Cranberry juice: 300–500 mL per day

Arctostaphylos uva ursi (Bearberry): *Uva ursi*'s main constituent arbutin is a strong urinary antiseptic. Arbutin is rapidly hydrolyzed to hydroquinone giving the herb a strong antiseptic effect (best in alkaline urine), especially against *E. coli*.[10] The safety of hydroquinone has been questioned and should not be used long term, however the amounts of free hydroquinone are miniscule to non-existent.[11] A double-blind placebo controlled study testing the prophylactic impact of *uva ursi*, showed no recurrence in women taking standardized *uva ursi*.[12] *Uva ursi* extract, corilagin, may enhance the efficacy of antibiotics such as oxacillin and other beta-lactam antibiotics against antibiotic resistant bacteria such as methicillin-resistant *Staphylococcus aureus* (MRSA).[13]

- **Dosing:**
  - Dried leaves: 1.5–4 g (1–2 tsp) three times per day
  - Tincture (1:5): 4–6 mL (1–1.5 tsp) three times per day
  - Solid extract (10% arbutin): (250–500 mg) three times per day

    H. Canadensis (Goldenseal) root: Goldenseal contains berberine, which is among the most effective herbal antimicrobials, like *uva ursi*, works best in alkaline urine. Two *in vitro* studies exhibited anti-adhesive effects of berberine on uropathogenic bacteria *E. coli* and *Streptococcus pyogenes*.[14]

- **Dosing:**
  - Dried root or tea: 1–2 g three times per day
  - Tincture (1:5): 4–6 mL (1–1.5 tsp) three times per day

Alkaline or acidic urine?

Benefits of alkalinizing urine seems to show promise with the use of citrate salts (potassium and sodium citrate). A group of women with a suspected UTI were given 4 g of sodium citrate every 8 hours for 48 hours. 80% of the 64 women showed symptom relief, indicating increasing urine pH may provide relief until a culture is obtained. Results varied with the women with abacterial symptomology.[15]

Overactive Bladder (OAB)

OAB presents with the main symptom of urgency, which often, but not necessarily, includes frequency, nocturia, and incontinence. OAB significantly impacts on patient quality of life, yet naturopathic modalities certainly help improve OAB symptoms and impact on daily functions.

Diet and lifestyle

Many of the current studies connecting food and OAB are slim yet two longitudinal studies done by Dallosso *et al.* investigated the impact of diet on OAB in men and women. Potatoes were found to be associated with OAB in men, yet surprisingly, beer independent of total alcohol content, was negatively associated. Studies have not shown significant correlations between OAB and alcohol intake. In women, bread, chicken and total vegetables (individual groups of vegetables such as legumes and brassicas did not show any significance) significantly reduced the risk of OAB onset, whereas carbonated beverages showed an increased risk.[16]

Phytoestrogens, in animal studies, have shown to increase the collagen to smooth muscle ratio, which theoretically may increase resting bladder pressure. The SWAN study investigated 2,721 women's phytoestrogen diet intake. Results showed no significant correlation with phytoestrogen intake and urinary incontinence.[17]

Several large studies have shown positive correlations of caffeine intake with incontinence and urgency. One dose-dependent study indicated caffeine intake $\geq 204\,mg/day$ to correlate with incontinence.[18] However, there is no evidence indicating caffeine may progress OAB.[19] In contrast, a large population Swedish study showed high tea consumption to increase the risk of OAB, whereas coffee, which is higher in caffeine, decreased risk.[20]

Body weight is a large factor in OAB, where obese and overweight women show a very high correlation with OAB and increased risk of OAB onset. Physical activity also played a role, as men and women who were more physically active showed a decreased risk of OAB onset.[16]

Dietetic and Lifestyle Approach

- Weight management to reduce body mass index (BMI) and %Total body fat
- Increased physical activity to 30 minutes 4–5 times per week
- Increase vegetable and lean meat intake such as chicken, turkey, fish
- Avoidance of alcohol, caffeine, smoking,[16] and carbonated beverages
- Eliminate aspartame

Nutraceuticals

Vitamin C studies have produced uncertain results with the impact on urinary urgency and frequency. The role of vitamin C in OAB is unclear, however, a large study showed vitamin C supplementation to increase frequency and urgency, whereas dietary vitamin C did not.[21] Another study supports these findings with decreased storage symptoms and urgency in men and women.[22]

- **Dosing:**
  - o Encourage foods high in vitamin C, but avoid vitamin C supplementation

Vitamin D has shown great promise, especially with lower urinary tract symptoms (LUTS) and OAB. A large study of 6,371 women showed a decrease in OAB onset with increased vitamin D intake.[23] 6000IU of a vitamin D analogue, elocalcitriol, showed a decrease in urinary frequency and patient perception of bladder condition (PPBC).[24]

- **Dosing:**
  - o Encourage patients to obtain their vitamin D from sunlight or consume dietary sources such as egg yolks, cod liver oil, and wild salmon

o Supplemental: At minimum 1,000 IU/day and up to 6,000 IU/ day with meals adjusted to optimal 25-(OH)D blood serum levels of approximately 50 nmol/L

Magnesium acts as a smooth muscle relaxant which explains its therapeutic effect in OAB possibly by decreasing detrusor activity. Magnesium hydroxide in levels as low as 146 mg were shown to significantly reduce urgency in women.

• **Dosing:**

o Magnesium hydroxide* — 146–246 mg twice daily (*Although the research used Mg hydroxide, magnesium citrate, and glycinate are more bioavailable and better assimilated. Therefore, it is recommended to use citrate or glycinate.)

Botanicals

Gosha-jinki-gan (GJG) is a Chinese herbal formula of 10 different blended herbs. In early animal studies, GJG decreased detrusor contraction in dogs and decreased spinal k opioid receptors in mice to decrease bladder sensation and frequency. A 44, women trial showed 7.5 g/d of GJG to improve International Prostate Symptom Score (IPSS), quality of life and daytime frequency,[25] with 9% of patients having adverse effects (AE). A second study of 30 men showed 2.5 g three times daily of GJG to significantly reduce IPSS, OABSS and improve quality of life score with three patients showing nausea, diarrhea and frequency.[26]

• **Dosing:**

o 2.5 g, three times daily

Ganoderma lucidum (GL), also known as Red Reishi, was tested at 0.6 mg, 6 mg, and 60 mg daily in 50 men. All three doses were shown to significantly improve IPSS scores by 3.22 over eight weeks, with no changes in PSA, residual urine and prostate volume without AE.[27]

- **Dosing:**

  o 0.6–60 mg daily

Pumpkin seed oil (*Cucurbita maxima*) was tested among 25 male and 20 female volunteers with OAB. Subjects consumed 10 g of *C. maxima* oil daily for 12 weeks. Results showed significant decreases in OABSS, daytime frequency, nighttime frequency, urgency and urgency incontinence without AE.[28]

- **Dosing:**

  o 10 mg of oil daily

Male Pelvic Pain

IC/PBS predominantly occurs in women, it is possible in men. However, a more common cause of pelvic pain in men is Chronic Prostatitis/Chronic Pelvic Pain Syndrome (CP/CPPS). Approximately, 2 million men per year seek help for CP/CPPS, therefore leading to a great necessity for treatment. The medical treatment for CP/CPPS currently is symptom specific, however, a naturopathic approach is whole body as CP/CPPS begins outside the prostate.

Diet

The impact of diet on CP/CPPS is often disregarded in medicine as possible triggers and cause of this condition. Few studies have shown a correlation with food sensitivities which worsened CP/CPPS symptoms, often targeted to a select set of foods including citrus fruits, coffee (caffeinated and decaffeinated), caffeinated beverages (tea, soda), dark and milk chocolate candy and spicy foods (chili, cayenne, etc.).[29] This also correlated with increased CPSI and OSPI scores. Psyllium fiber may palliate symptoms.

The coexistence of IBS and CP/CPPS has been seen clinically and also in the literature. Oftentimes these patients experience leaky gut syndrome (hyperpermeable intestines), predisposing them to increased risk of food sensitivities and intolerances, which supports the correlation of food irritants and CP/CPPS.

The goal in these patients is to avoid hyperallergenic foods including dairy (casein/whey), gluten and soy. Food sensitivity tests, testing for IgG and IgE are beneficial in exposing and eliminating antigenic foods. An elimination diet is less costly option allowing men to remove select foods and reintroduce them identifying possible trigger foods.

Omega-3 oils: EPA and DHA

The benefits of omega-3 oils is far-reaching, and their most useful indication would be for chronic inflammation.[30] CP is a chronic inflammatory disease which would see great benefit from daily fish oil intake.

- **Dosing:**
  - 4–6 g daily of EPA and DHA total

Nutraceuticals

DIM (Diindolemethane)

This compound found in many cruciferous vegetables has been shown to promote healthy prostate function and cellular health[31] which may prove beneficial in an irritated prostate. Additionally, it promotes the production of estrogens into 2-series which are less potent that than 4 and 16 series estrogens.

- **Dosing:**
  - 100 mg/daily

Pollen extract

Compared to placebo, Pollen extract significantly reduced pain and symptom, improved QOL in men and resulted in overall favorable results including improved urine flow and improved DRE in men with CP/CPPS.[32]

- **Dosing:**

  o 500 mg/daily

Pygeum (*Prunus africana*)

Pygeum has historically been used for urinary condition, yet for CP has shown promise in reducing chronic prostatitis symptoms including decreased sexual function and also improved QOL and urinary parameters.[33]

- **Dosing:**

  o 100–200 mg/day

Naturopathic modalities approach patients from multiple angles including multiple treatment options. One excellent example of this is the combination of Saw palmetto 160 mg (*Serona repens*), Stinging Nettle 120 mg (*Urtica dioca radix*), Curcumin 200 mg (from Turmeric, *Curcuma longa*) and Quercetin 100 mg. This combination was tested in men with chronic bacterial prostatitis along with 600 mg prulifloxacin in two groups on men, Group A receiving the antibiotic with the four herbs and Group B only the antibiotic. 90% of the men in Group A had resolution of symptoms without recurrence within six months, whereas only 27% of men in the antibiotic only group showed resolution and two men had recurrence within six months.[34] This study indicates the promising benefits of integrative medicine and the ability of these four herbs to prevent chronic prostatitis. These herbs have also been tested independently each showing promising benefits in treating CP/CPPS, and Quercetin in particular may lower Chronic Prostatitis Index and IPSS within one month. Green tea catechin (EGCG) has also shown similar benefits in enhancing antibiotic use in prostatitis.[35]

- **Dosing:**

  o Saw palmetto 160–320 mg, Nettle root 120–240 mg, Curcumin 200–500 mg, Quercetin 100–500 mg
  o Green tea: 4–5 cups daily (Decaffeinated may be used to avoid irritation)

Vitamin D3

Vitamin D3 has a multitude of benefits especially considering its prominent deficiency in the male urological population.[36] This hormone has exemplified significant benefit in treatment of other prostate conditions including BPH and LUTS without any serious adverse effects. Therefore, it would be prudent to optimized vitamin D levels above 50 ng/mL.

- **Dosing:**

  o 1,000–5,000 IU Vitamin D_3 (Cholecalciferol) daily with food

Zinc

Researchers have found lower concentrations of zinc in men who have prostatitis than in healthy controls, indicating that zinc supplements may be recommended for men with prostatitis.[37] Additional levels of 220 mg/day of Zn reduced symptoms and pain score in men with CP/CPPS, however, caution must be taken with such a large dose.[38]

- **Dosing:**

  o 30–60 mg daily for six months then reduce to 30 mg daily

Probiotics

Urethral dysbacteriosis caused by excessive antibiotic use is a possible cause of CP/CPPS.[39] In men experiencing Chronic Bacterial Prostatitis and IBS, combination of VSL#3 with rifaximin reduced CP symptoms and prevented progression in men with cured chronic bacteria prostatitis and IBS.[40]

- **Dose:**
  - o 50–100 million CFU three times daily

Female Pelvic Pain

A Therapeutic Approach to Interstitial Cystitis and Painful Bladder Syndrome (IC/PBS)

IC/PBS is non-infectious bladder inflammation that is characterized by CPP (suprapubic, pelvic, and abdominal) and urinary urgency and frequency without incontinence. IC is often a diagnosis of exclusion, yet naturopathic modalities have shown some promise in treating patients to enhance quality of life and reduce symptomology.

Diet and lifestyle

Although a definitive cause of IC/PBS has not been established, the theory of a dysregulated bladder urothelial barrier, specifically the glycosaminoglycan (GAG) layer of the urothelium, proposes there may be some innocuous substances allowed to penetrate the typically well-regulated epithelium causing usually benign stimuli to become irriating.[4] This theory is supported by the potassium sensitivity test (PST) which may indicate a defective bladder lining with increased permeability.[41]

Several studies have concluded on the strong connection between specific comestibles and IC/PBS. The consensus shows caffeinated beverages/foods, alcohol, artificial sweeteners, carbonated beverages (soda), grapefruit juice, citrus fruits and spicy foods (chili, hot peppers) exacerbated symptoms in patients with IC/PBS.[84] Other foods promoting relief are psyllium, baking soda, calcium glycerophosphate, docusate, polycarbophil, and water.[42]

An elimination diet may identify the actual offenders worsening IC/PBS. For two weeks, the patient will abstain from common food allergens gluten, dairy, common offenders, and record symptoms. After two weeks, the patient will then reintroduce one eliminated food type at a time to record any adverse symptoms, waiting three days before adding an additional eliminated food. Elimination diets allow accurate identification of problematic foods in helping the patient avoid pain and discomfort.

The coexistence of Irritable Bowel Syndrome and IC/PBS is irrefutable,[43] yet a causative association has not been established. Some theories propose 'cross-talk' occurs between organs as stimuli from one organ may impact another. Noxious stimuli may irritate colonocytes, via mast cells, directly irritating bladder sensory C-fibers.[4]

Botanicals

A Chinese herbal tea containing *Cornus, gardenia, curculigo,* rhubarb, *Psoralea,* and *Rehmannia* reduced pain in 61% of patients within four weeks and an additional 22% of subjects reported decreased pain within three months.[44]

Centella asiatica (Gotu Kola): Gotu kola works by tonifying connective tissue and especially strengthens smooth muscle of the urinary system, thus possibly enhancing the function and integrity of urothelium.[45]

- **Dose:**
  - Tea: three times per day
  - Capsules: 1–4g, three times per day
  - Tincture (1:2 w:v 30% alcohol): 1.5–3 mL, three times per day
  - Extract (standardized: 40% asiaticoside, 29–30% Asiatic acid, 29–30% madecassic acid and 1–2% madecassoside): 50–250 mg, 2–3 times per day

Equisetum arvense (Horsetail): This astringent herb has high silica content and has been used traditionally to heal GU conditions.[46]

- **Dose**[92]:
  - ○ Standardized dose (10–15% silica): 300 mg three times per day
  - ○ Tea: 2–3 tsp of infused herb, three times per day
  - ○ Tincture (1:5): 1–4 mL, three times per day

Nutraceuticals

L-Arginine:

This popular amino acid produces nitric oxide (NO) when catalyzed by nitric oxide synthetase (NOS) leading to multiple benefits including smooth muscle relaxation.[47] L-arginine use for IC/PBS is arguable and sometimes shown to have no benefit,[48] however, some research shows low NOS in IC patients. A randomized double-blind trial showed 1.5 g of L-arginine daily for three months to reduce the symptoms in 29% (6 of 21) of the arginine treatment group and only 8% (2 of 21) of the placebo group. A Likert scale showed improvement in the arginine group with decreased pain intensity, decreased pain frequency and improved urgency, yet an intention-to-treat analysis showed no benefit.[49]

- **Dose:**
  - ○ L-Arginine: 750 mg, two times per day

Quercetin

This fat soluble flavonoid is found in citrus fruits, olive oil, onions, apples, capers, tea, and red wine. Quercetin is known to inhibit mast cell histamine release, along with acting as an anti-inflammatory. One study showed 500 mg of quercetin twice daily for four weeks was able to reduce the global assessment of pain (Likert scale), along with a significant improvement in the O'Leary Sant Symptom and problem indices.[50]

- **Dose:**

  o Quercetin: 500 mg, two times per day

Urge Incontinence

Protocols treating urge incontinence, where the need to urinate is unable to be restrained, are similar to those used to treat OAB (see OAB treatments).

Vitamin B12 deficiency must be considered as a possible cause of urge incontinence, as it may lead to detrusor underactivity.[51] Serum B12 levels are not a complete representation of B12 status, as methylmalonic acid should also be tested.

- **Dose:**

  o Sublingual Methylcobalamin: 1,000–5,000 mcg/day
  o Intramuscular methylcobalamin injection: 1,000 mgcg

Stress Incontinence

Stress urinary incontinence (SUI) is caused by increased intra-abdominal pressure, often occurring with sneezing, laughing, coughing, etc.

Obesity

With a correlation between visceral adipose index, body mass index (BMI) and SUI,[52] weight management is an effective approach in reducing SUI.[53] Reducing central adiposity will reduce pressure on the bladder thus resolving symptoms. Methods in doing so are discussed in the following section.

Diet and Lifestyle

The major dietary goal is to reduce irritation on the bladder and pelvic muscles. Common identified irritants to avoid include alcohol, smoking, carbonated drinks, and saturated fat. Vitamin B12, cholesterol, saturated fat, and zinc intakes are all positively associated with SUI, of which red meat is an excellent source.[16] Therefore, red meat consumption may be a possible irritant as well.

As mentioned in the previous sections, minimizing blood glucose through a low glycemic diet limits inflammation and irritation. Women with diabetes are more prone to SUI, thus indicating a sugar-control diet may be helpful in reducing symptoms,[54] which may be achieved with a low glycemic/low carb dietary approach.

Coffee, caffeinated soft drinks and tea should be minimized. Caffeine intake greater than 169 mg/day (which is 1–2 cups of coffee) is associated with SUI compared to lower intakes. Caffeine may irritate the bladder, as seen in OAB and IC, therefore it would be prudent to minimize exposure in individuals with SUI.

Benign Prostatic Hyperplasia (BPH)

Diet and lifestyle

An ideal goal for men with BPH would be to reduce total body weight optimally through reducing calories and increasing protein intake from vegetables and cold-water fish sources, as these have been shown to decrease BPH risk,[55] possibly by reducing 5α reductase activity.[56] A high BMI, hyperinsulinemia, and hyperglycemia increases sympathetic tone and promotes prostate smooth muscle contraction,[57] therefore a low carb/low glycemic/high protein diet may reduce symptoms.

Total fat intake, not specific to any particular type (saturated, mono- and poly-unsaturated) is correlated with BPH.[55] Cardiovascular (CV) disease risk is linked to BPH/LUTS suggesting protecting the CV system will also protect against BPH,[58] including omega-3 oils. Lipid oxidation may promote the progression of BPH, and therefore perhaps it is lipid oxidation not necessarily the fats promoting BPH.[59]

Therapeutic approach

- Reduce body weight, total body fat percent and increase physical activity
- Focus on moderate protein intake with emphasis on vegetables and cold-water fish sources
- Limit meat, butter, margarine, caffeine, alcohol intake

  o Focus on grass-fed, wild, hormone-free foods

- Increase fruit, vegetable and soy intake while limiting carbohydrate intake to low glycemic sources and limiting dairy intake

Nutraceuticals

Zinc

Zinc, found to be low in BPH tissue,[60] may reduce 5α reductase activity[61] and prolactin levels,[62] which may indicate its benefit in reducing BPH size, symptoms, and reduce risk.[63]

- **Dose:**

  o 30–45 mg/day (Zn picolinate) the reduce to 15–40 mg/day after six months

  *Monitor copper status, Zn may deplete copper levels

Amino acids — Glycine, glutamic acid, alanine

These three amino acids at doses of 200 mg/day each have shown to palliate BPH symptoms of nocturia, urgency, frequency, and delayed micturition.

Vitamin D3 (Cholecalciferol)

Vitamin D intake (dietary and supplementary) at doses greater than 440IU tends to decrease BPH risk.[64] At doses up to 6000IU, prostate growth can be arrested but without change in symptoms or uroflowmetry.[65] Mechanistically, vitamin D3 binds Vitamin D Receptors on the prostate and bladder inhibiting intraprostatic growth factors downstream and androgen response, along with exerting anti-inflammatory activities.

- **Dose:**
  - 2000–5000IU daily with food

Female Sexual Dysfunction

Approximately 40% of women experience low sexual desire.[66] Low female libido can have numerous physical, psychological, emotional, and social impacts on a woman's life. Not many pharmaceuticals are designed for female libido, but several naturopathic remedies show promise.

Female androgens, estrogens and the connection with diminished libido has been questioned, yet sexual dysfunction is multifactorial and often not limited to one variable (see Figure 1).[68] Not to be ignored, low fluctuating testosterone and decreased DHEA are evident in pre- and post-menopausal women experiencing low sexual desire,[69] with lowered DHEA evident also in younger women (18–45 years). Because DHEA is a precursor to both T and

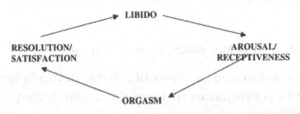

Figure 1:   Relationship between female libido, arousal, orgasm, and satisfaction.[67]

estrogen, it may promote sexual function in hypoestrogenic women, particularly perimenopausal women, as estrogen impacts vaginal lubrication, vascular and muscular integrity of urogenital organs, mood, sleep and cognitive function holistically impacting sexual desire directly and indirectly.[70] This may indicate the benefit of intravaginal and oral DHEA on female sexual function.[71] Androgens, which may be increased by providing precursor DHEA, are responsible for psychosexual stimulation, increased genitalia sensitivity and increased sexual gratification, all of which are connected to libido.

• **Dose:**

  o 5–50 mg DHEA daily, beginning at 5 mg and increasing until improvement

In younger women with normal hormonal levels, several solutions exist with minimal to no impact on androgens or estrogens. Within four weeks, a combination of l-arginine, *Gingko biloba, Panax ginseng,* and *Turnera aphrodesiaca* (found in product Arginmax) were shown to significantly improve sex life including sexual desire, vaginal dryness, orgasm, and sexual frequency without any impact on hormonal levels.[72]

• **Dose:**

  o Six capsules daily — divided throughout the day

Magnolia bark (*Magnolia officianlis*) when added to a combination of magnesium, soy isoflavone and *L. sporogenes* was shown to significantly improve female libido, reduce vaginal dryness, reduce dyspareunia and reduce irritability in menopausal women with no impact on hormonal levels.[73]

• **Dose:**

  o 60 mg/daily of Magnolia bark

Menopausal related libido loss can be relieved with the use of Pycnogenol. This extract has been shown to reduce vaginal dryness, improve libido and increase sexual behavior within eight weeks without any impact on hormonal levels.[74]

- **Dose:**
  - o 100 mg/daily

Maca

Of all the herbs, maca root has shown great promise clinically in enhancing female libido. Best yet without any impact on hormonal levels enhancing its safety. Maca has even been shown to improve sexual function in SSRI-induced sexual dysfunction and also increase libido.[75]

- **Dose:**
  - o 3 g daily

The psychosocial relationship is not to be ignored, and the impact of a healthy sexual relationship extends far beyond the bedroom. Patients may require counseling in scenarios that may assist their relationship and improve their intimacy, as their mood outside the bedroom impacts interpretations of sexual experiences.

Female Orgasm Disorder

The treatments for female libido disorders may also be applicable to female orgasm disorder. Especially when deficient, estrogenic and androgenic impact on genitalia impacts sexual response, sexual gratification, libido, all of which impact orgasmic capacity.[75]

A topical treatment containing borage seed oil, evening primrose oil, *Angelica sinensis* extract (dong quai), *Coleus forskohlii*, theobromine, and vitamin C and E was shown clinically to improve symptoms in women with sexual arousal and orgasm disorders.[76]

- **Dose:**
  - Apply topically 5–10 minutes before intercourse

Male Sexual Dysfunction

Erectile dysfunction (ED) is multifactorial and often coexisting with psychiatric (depression) disorders, relationship/sexual partner issues and misconceptions of sex. ED may also exist as organic (neurogenic, hormonal or most commonly vascular in nature) or mixed psychogenic-organic. The 'artery size' hypothesis suggests men with coronary artery disease will report ED before CAD is identified,[77] therefore it is essential to asses CV health in men with ED (Figure 2).

L-Arginine

L-Arginine (Arg) is a precursor in the synthesis of NO catalyzed by endothelial NO synthase (NOS) which works to relax endothelial tissue and enhance blood flow. As measured in by the International Index of Erectile Function (IIEF), Erection Hardness Score (EHS) and ED Inventory of Treatment Satisfaction, 5.2 g l-Arg with 200 mg of adenosine monophosphate was shown to enhance erectile function within 1–2 hours of intercourse.[79] 6 mg of Arg with 6 mg of Yohimbe may improve ED within 2 hours.[80] The ratio of asymmetrical dimethylarginine (ADMA), an inhibitor of NOS to Arg (Arg/ADMA), was lower in men with artiogenic ED indicating Arg may play a significant role in arteriogenic ED.Paroni.[81]

- **Dosing:**
  - 3–6 g/day

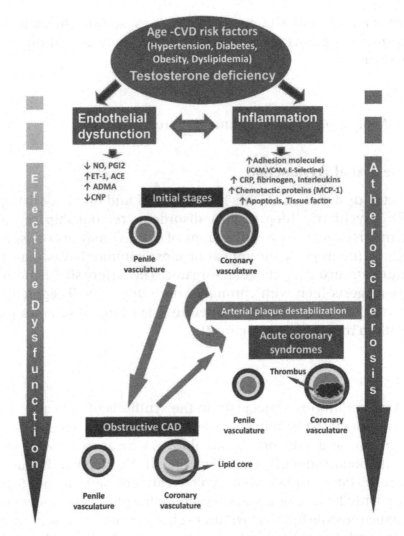

Figure 2:   Pathogenesis of ED and relation to atherosclerosis.[78]

L-Citrulline

L-cirtrulline (Cit) acts as an L-Arg precursor leading to a sustained increase in NO. The half-life of L-Arg *in vivo* is not sustained and therefore L-Cit provides a prolonged increased in NO resulting in enhanced endothelial function, including penile tissue.[82]

- **Dosing:**

  o 1.5 g/day

Epimedium and icariin

Epimedium spp. works similar to common ED drugs. The constituent icariin acts as a phosphodiesterase-5 inhibitor supporting levels of cGMP in penile corpus cavernosum. This results in healthy erections even at doses as low as 1 mg/kg of body weight.[83]

- **Dosing:**

  o 50–150 mg Icariin daily (*Epimedium* standardized to icariin)

Resveratrol

This antioxidant is common to most Americans as the healthy ingredient in red wine, enhances corpus cavernosum relaxation by endogenous vasodilation, enhances NOS and acetylcholine induced vasodilation. The vasorelaxation induced by resveratrol is systemic and may benefit atherosclerotic conditions.[83]

- **Dosing:**

  o 200–300 mg/day

Rhodiola

The multifactorial impact on ED including psychogenic aspect of ED need not be ignored. This adaptogen has been shown to reduce fatigue, impact stress response and improve immune function in stressful situations, making it essential to reduce stress, anxiety and help psychogenic/mixed ED.[84]

- **Dosing:**

  o 250–750 mg/day

Pomegranate

This prostate-nourishing antioxidant is rich in anthocyanin — a powerful flavonoid that enhances erection-stimulating NO bioavailability by inhibiting NO breakdown, while promoting optimal penile blood flow by decreasing penile tissue fibrosis. Pomegranate may be able to facilitate firm erections and enhance sexual performance in men with both CV and erectile function concerns — two challenges that often present simultaneously.[84]

- Dosing
  - 8 o' pomegranate juice daily

DHEA

Testing DHEA-S levels may be prudent in identifying the underlying cause without an organic or psychogenic cause. Studies have shown correlations with low DHEA and ED, and several clinical studies have shown improvement in penetration and maintenance of an erection at doses of 50 mg of DHEA in men as young as 40 (no data on men <40).[85] Androgens are responsible for psychosexual stimulation, increased genitalia sensitivity and increased sexual gratification[86] which may enhance erections.

Exercise

This often overlooked lifestyle change can have tremendous benefits in CV health. Men with CV risk factors show decreased ED risk with high intensity exercise.[87]

Dietary approach

The connection between chronic disease and inflammation is not to be ignored, with a high carbohydrate/high glycemic diet promoting a pro-inflammatory state and contributes to daily inflammation. A low-glycemic diet will reduce atherosclerotic risk and risk of ED,[88] with a Mediterranean diet showing most benefit.[89] The risk of ED was also associated with higher HbA1c, commonly seen in high glycemic diets.[90]

Disorders of Male Orgasm, Low Libido, and Low Testosterone

The interplay of low testosterone (low T), low libido and male orgasm disorders are independent conditions but interrelated and often treated together. Naturopathic modalities focus on whole body health and therefore focusing on the whole individual often resolves multiple conditions as a pure result of proper communication and function of the sex organs and the body.

Male Orgasm disorder is often related to organic vasogenic ED, as decreased blood flow to the penis impacts rigidity, erection time and ejaculation which ultimately manifests as premature ejaculation or male orgasm dysfunction.[91]

The pregnenolone/cortisol steal is often seen clinically and is independent of adrenal enzymatic deficiency. In chronically stressed patients, pregnenolone production is shunted to cortisol and away from androgens, resulting in low T and low androgen production.

DHEA

This testosterone precursor declines with age in men. DHEA supplementation may increase testosterone levels, with benefits seen in older men (45+) and even younger men in their 20s, without deleterious effects.[92] Some studies have conflicting findings,[93] yet it is essential to consider androgen levels, SHBG, estradiol, along with thyroid hormone and stress as these all impact DHEA and androgen metabolism.

- **Dose:**
  - 25–100 mg before bed, adjusted to DHEA-S, estrogen, and androgen levels

Tongkat Ali (*Eurycoma longifolia*)

Tongkat has limited but promising research exposing its benefits on increasing testosterone, yet only two studies have shown such benefit in hypogonadal men. Tongkat has also been shown to lower SHBG which can effectively increase free T.[94]

- **Dose:**
  - o 100–200 mg/daily

Maca root (*Lepidium meyenii*)

This Peruvian root does not impact androgens or LH/FSH in men, but it does improve libido and sexual desire in men independent of hormonal levels.[95]

- **Dose:**
  - o 3 g/daily

Ashwagandha (*Withania sominifera*)

This adaptogen is classically known to assist with stress and anxiety, yet research has shown it to significantly improve testosterone levels by impacting LH levels in infertile men. It also lowers cortisol levels which play an important role is the 'pregnenolone steal' factor.[96]

- **Dose:**
  - o 600–700 mg divided daily

Mucuna pruriens (*Dopa bean*)

This plant often used for its L-dopa constituent has also been shown in two double-blind studies to statistically increase testosterone and improve fertility in infertile men. Like *ashwagandha*, it may reduce cortisol, which plays into the stress factor.[97]

- **Dose:**

  o 800 mg to –5 g daily

Nettle root (*Urtica dioica radix*)

Although not directly increasing T, nettle root inhibits SHBG from binding bioavailable T and also inhibits aromatase resulting in more T and less estradiol.[98]

- **Dose:**

  o 300–900 mg divided daily

Tribulus terrestris

The increase in T from *Tribulus* seems to be limited to animal studies and human studies have not shown significant enhancement in T levels.[99] A mild benefit was seen in erection and male libido.[99] The research does not support *Tribulus* to assist in testosterone, libido, and male orgasm.[100]

Zinc

This element has gained a reputation for being essential for men, with multiple research studies backing that claim. Zinc has been shown to preserve and enhance T levels and thyroid hormones (which are integral in optimizing testicular and adrenal function) in men.[101]

- **Dose:**

  o 15–30 mg daily — preferably as zinc picolinate

Diet and weight loss

Fat cells aromatize testosterone into estrogen, therefore weight loss and fat loss in particular in men with high body fat will reduce this conversion and improve T levels.[102] A low glycemic diet minimizes insulin release and also reduces eicosanoid (PGE2) production. Insulin upregulates delta-5 reductase increasing production of PGE2, which may increase aromatase activity.[103] Omega-3 fats and poly and mono-unsaturated fats will reduce PGE2 production and provide healthy lipids for T production.

Endocrine disruptors

Endocrine disruptors including DES, BPA, DDT, PCB, Genistein, and Dioxins have been shown to impact male fertility and reproductive organs. These constituents are commonly found in plastics and large fish from contaminated waters.[104] It is essential to minimize these exposures as they are often dismissed through adulthood.[105] Lead damages Leydig cells and may be a hidden cause of hypogonadism and low libido.[106]

Kidney stones

Kidney stones (Nephrolithiasis) are commonly asymptomatic until there is an acute onset of symptoms. They typically present as calcium stones, uric acid stones or struvite stones, all of which respond well to naturopathic protocols.

Calcium stones

Dietary changes can have one of the most profound impacts in preventing and reducing kidney stone development. Leafy green consumption, increased fiber and complex carbohydrates were associated with decreased stone formation and decreased calcium excretion.[107] Soft drinks, alcohol, fructose (sports drinks, juices, etc.) and refined carbohydrates (pasta, rice, sweets, white bread, etc.) were all correlated with increased calcium excretion[108] and increased stone formation.[109] In fact, abstaining from soft drinks and fructose reduced stone formation.[108] Refined carbohydrates and sugar elicit a strong insulin increase shown to cause hypercalciuria, thus are considered high-risk factors for stone formation.[110] Sodium (also found in soft drinks) increases calcium excretion and reduces protective urinary citrate concentrations thus promoting stone formation.[111]

Water, as simple as it seems, at 2 L per day dilutes urine and multiple randomized trials exhibited up to a 60% decrease in stone formation.[112]

A complete dietary approach would include

- Reduction in soft drinks, fructose, refined/simple carbohydrates
- Low sodium diet <2 g day
- Increased water intake to 2 L/day
- Increased consumption of leafy greens, fibrous fruits and vegetables, and complex carbohydrates
- Avoidance of oxalate containing foods (black tea, cocoa, spinach, parsley, nuts, and cranberries.)

Nutraceuticals

Magnesium (Mg)

Multiple studies have shown Mg to increase solubility of oxalate stones and prevent precipitation. Vitamin B6 (Pyridoxine) has been shown to greatly enhance these effects especially in recurrent stone formation, which is likely due to B6 acting as a cofactor in oxalate-metabolizing transaminases.[113]

Potassium citrate, calcium citrate, and most helpful magnesium citrate have shown to reduce urinary calcium oxalate concentration and retard crystal growth.[114]

- **Dosing:**
    - Magnesium citrate: 600 mg/day and Vitamin B6: 25 mg/day

Calcium

Low calcium diets, contrary to common medical advice, are correlated with increase in stone formation, and in doses from 300 to

1,000 mg daily may prevent calcium excretion and stone formation.[115] Excess calcium may deplete magnesium thus it is prudent to supplement both. Vitamin D in excess can cause hypercalcemia, however recent studies have not shown a correlation with calcium stones and in fact should not be withheld in those with calcium stones and D3 deficiency.[116]

- **Dosing:**

  o 300–1,000 mg/day of Calcium citrate

Vitamin K

Vitamin K, common in green leafy vegetables, is essential to form gamma-carboxygluatmic acid, which acts as a urinary oxalate inhibitor. Vitamin K insufficiency may explain oxalate stone formation, and also the decreased incidence of stone formation in vegetarians.[117]

- **Dosing:**

  o 2 mg/day (preferably as MK-7)

Inositol hexaphosphate (IP6, Phytic Acid)

This compound commonly found in whole grains, cereals, nuts, legumes, and seeds has been shown to significantly reduce calcium oxalate crystals within 15 days.[118]

- **Dosing:**

  o 120 mg/day

Uric acid stones

Reducing purine rich foods is essential in treating uric acid stones. These foods have shown a direct linear correlation with urinary uric acid.[119] Increased vegetable intake, even with meat consumption has shown to lower uric acid stone formation.[120]

Blackcurrant juice and leafy greens increase urinary pH, reducing the risk of Uric acid stone formation. Bicarbonate and citrate will help reduce uric acid crystallization.[121]

Foods rich in purines

High Purine Foods

- All meats: Organ meats, beef, lamb, pork
- Seafood: Including shellfish
- Yeast and yeast extracts
- Beer and other alcoholic drinks
- Beans, peas, lentils, oatmeal, spinach, asparagus, cauliflower, mushrooms

Nutraceuticals

Folic acid is an essential nutrient in scavenging purines which will be metabolized in uric acid. Therefore, folic acid may prevent this process.

- **Dose:**
  o 5 mg/day

Cystine stones

Cystine stones are often an inherited condition which can be assisted with reduction in methionine rich foods including soy, wheat, dairy, milk, fish, meat, lima beans, garbanzo beans, and all nuts (excluding coconut, hazelnut, and sunflower seeds).

Struvite stones

Struvite stones form in an alkaline urine and are potentiated by urea-splitting organisms. To reduce urinary pH, cranberry juice daily may be helpful.[121]

- **Dosing**

  o 100% Cranberry juice — 11 oz/day

Vitamin C

There is conflicting evidence on the benefits and detriments of vitamin C on oxalate excretion. Some studies have shown no increased risk, whereas others have shown increase urinary oxalates[122] with Ester-C showing a minimal oxalate excretion.[123] It would be most safe to avoid vitamin C in patients with a history of nephrolithiasis, and Ester-C should be of choice if vitamin C is to be used.

Heavy metals

Cadmium serum levels have been correlated with a 40% increase risk of stone formation, therefore it would be prudent to test using hair analysis or serum to rule out possible metal toxicity.[124]

Bowel and GI Disturbances

In the treatment of OAB, IC/PBS and CP/CPPS, it is absolutely necessary to be aware these conditions often coexist or precede gastrointestinal (GI) disorders such as IBS and IBD. GI symptoms may be ignored or confused with GU condtions,[125] and are not to be dismissed as independent conditions.

Naturopathy observes the patient as a whole without isolating conditions therefore in treating the gut, GU conditions are also addressed. Treatments specific to OAB, IC/PBS, CP/CPPS are found in their respective section, however, here a comprehensive approach is taken.

An explicit correlation between specific food allergens and IC/PBS, CP/CPPS exists in men and women (see Table 1 in IC/PBS).[16] Increased gut permeability (Leaky Gut) may allow food allergens to by-pass enterocyte tight-junctions and cause systemic immune responses impacting GU and GI afferent and efferent nerves.[126] Clinically, eliminating foods such as gluten, soy, and dairy (casein and whey) results in symptom relief and pauses progression.

Table 1. List of Common Offending Foods Known to Exacerbate IC/PBS Symptoms and a List of Foods Known to not Exacerbate IC/PBS Symptoms[4]

Common Offending Foods to IC/PBS	Least Offending Foods to IC/PBS
Tea (Caffeinated)	Milk, low fat, and whole
Carbonated beverage, Cola, and Non-Cola	
Diet carbonated beverage	Bananas
Carbonated beverage, caffeine-free	Blueberries
Beer	Honeydew melon
Wine, red, and white champagne	Pears
	Raisins
Grapefruit	Watermelon
Lemon	
Orange	Broccoli
Pineapple	Brussels Sprouts
Cranberry juice	Cabbage
Grapefruit juice	Cauliflower
Orange juice	Celery
Pineapple juice	Cucumber
	Mushrooms
Tomato	Peas
Tomato products	Radishes
Hot peppers	Squash
Spicy foods	Zucchini
Chili	White potatoes
Horseradish	Sweet potatoes/Yams
Vinegar	
Monosodium glutamate	Chicken
	Eggs
NutraSweet	Turkey
Sweet'N Low	Beef
Equal (sweetener)	Pork
Saccharin	Lamb

(Continued)

Table 1.   (*Continued*)

Common Offending Foods to IC/PBS	Least Offending Foods to IC/PBS
	Shrimp
Mexican food	Tuna fish
Thai food	Salmon
Indian food	
	Oat
	Rice
	Pretzels
	Popcorn

Overactive sympathetic tone and a decreased parasympathetic tone decreases gastric secretions and slows peristalsis.[127] Calm eating hygiene involving unrushed eating with conscious chewing (20–25 chews) optimizes autonomic control of digestion. It would be naïve to believe this has no connection to OAB, IC and CP/CPPS, therefore, practicing stress reduction can provide substantial relief of GI and thus GU symptoms.

Ways to reduce stress include guided meditation (even 5 minutes), conscious breathing exercises and daily exercise. Herbs to reduce anxiety and promote relaxation include:

• Passion flower (*Passiflora incarnate*)
• Lavender oil (*Lavendula angustifolia*)
• Kava (*Piper methysticum*)

Constipation commonly is associated with OAB and LUTS, which are likely due to a faulty nervous cross-talk between organ systems.[128] In general, relief from constipation results in palliation of OAB and LUTS.[5]

Water

Without proper hydration, stools become dry and difficult to pass.

• **Dose:**

  o 2 L/day

Fiber

Fiber from chia, flax, and psyllium not only improves intestinal health by providing gut flora with nutrients but also helps loosen stool and improve transmit time.

- **Dose:**
  - o Begin with 20 g of fiber per day and slowly increase up to 30 g daily

Probiotics

The benefits of these gut friendly bacteria are becoming more prominent in research with multiple studies indicating they improve gut transit time, stool frequency and consistency.[129]

- **Dose:**
  - o 25 billion CFU probiotic two times daily with a light meal

Magnesium

Often used as a safe osmotic laxative to assist in constipation, it also exhibits systemic and GI spasmolytic. Therefore, it may also be used for detrusor instability and sensory urgency.[130]

- **Dose:**
  - o Magnesium Citrate 400–700 mg/daily (in divided doses)

References

1. Clearinghouse NKaUDI. Kidney and Urologic Diseases Statistics for the United States Kidney disease; 2007.
2. Gupta K, Scholes D and Stamm WE. Increasing prevalence of antimicrobial resistance among uropathogens causing acute uncomplicated cystitis in women. *J Am Med Assoc.* 1999;281: 736–738.
3. Sanchez A, Reeser JL, Lau HS, *et al.* Role of sugars in human neutrophilic phagocytosis. *Am J Clin Nutr.* 1973;26:1180–1184.

4. Friedlander JI, Shorter B and Moldwin RM. Diet and its role in interstitial cystitis/bladder pain syndrome (IC/BPS) and comorbid conditions. *BJU Int.* 2012;109:1584–1591.

5. Kranjčec B, Papeš D and Altarac S. d-mannose powder for prophylaxis of recurrent urinary tract infections in women: a randomized clinical trial. *World J Urol.* 2014;32:79–84.

6. Zafriri D, Ofek I, Adar R, Pocino M and Sharon N. Inhibitory Activity of Cranberry Juice on Adherence of Type 1 and Type P Fimbriated Escherichia coli to Eucaryotic Cells. *Antimicrob Agents Chemother.* 1989;33(1):92–98.

7. Papas PN, Brusch CA and Ceresia GC. Cranberry juice in the treatment of urinary tract infections. *Southwest Med.* 1966;47:17–20.

8. Avorn J, Monane M, JH G, RJ G, Choodnovskiy I and LA L. Reduction of bacteriuria and pyuria after ingestion of cranberry juice. *JAMA.* 1994;271:751–754.

9. Wang C, Fang C, Chen N, *et al.* Cranberry-containing products for prevention of urinary tract infections in susceptible populations: A systematic review and meta-analysis of randomized controlled trials. *Arch Intern Med.* 2012;172:988–996.

10. Frohne D. The urinary disinfectant effect of extract from leaves uva ursi. *Planta Med.* 1970;18:1–25.

11. Paper D, Koehler J and Franz G. Bioavailability of drug preparations containing a leaf extract of Arctostaphylos uva-ursi. *Planta Med.* 1993;3:63–66.

12. Larsson B, Jonasson A and Fianu S. Prophylactic effect of UVA-E in women with recurrent cystitis: A preliminary report. *Curr Ther Res.* 2014;53:441–443.

13. Shimizu M, Shiota S, Mizushima T, *et al.* Marked Potentiation of Activity of β-Lactams against Methicillin-Resistant Staphylococcus aureus by Corilagin. *Antimicrob Agents Chemother.* 2001;45;3198–3201.

14. Sun D, Abraham SN and Beachey EH. Influence of berberine sulfate on synthesis and expression of Pap fimbrial adhesin in uropathogenic Escherichia coli. *Antimicrob Agents Chemother.* 1988;32; 1274–1277.

15. Munday PE and Savage S. Cymalon in the management of urinary tract symptoms. *Genitourin Med.* 1990;66:461.

16. Dallosso HM, McGrother CW, Matthews RJ, Donaldson MMK and Group tLMRCIS. The association of diet and other lifestyle factors with overactive bladder and stress incontinence: a longitudinal study in women. *BJU Int.* 2003;92:69–77.

17. Waetjen LE, Katherine L, Sybil LC, Mei-Hua H, Ellen BG and Greendale GA. Relationship between dietary phytoestrogens and development of urinary incontinence in midlife women. *Menopause.* 2013;20(4):428–436.

18. Gleason JL, Richter HE, Redden DT, Goode PS, Burgio KL and Markland AD. Caffeine and urinary incontinence in US women. *Int Urogynecol J.* 2013;24:295–302.

19. Townsend MK, Resnick NM and Grodstein F. Caffeine intake and risk of urinary incontinence progression among women. *Obstet Gynecol.* 2012;19(5):950–957.

20. Tettamanti G, Altman D, Pedersen NL, Bellocco R, Milsom I and Iliadou AN. Effects of coffee and tea consumption on urinary incontinence in female twins. *BJOG.* 2011;118:806–812.

21. Maserejian NN, Giovannucci EL, McVary KT and McKinlay JB. Intakes of vitamins and minerals in relation to urinary incontinence, voiding, and storage symptoms in women: A cross-sectional analysis from the boston area community health survey. *Eur Urol.* 2011;59:1039–1047.

22. Curto TM, Giovannucci EL, McKinlay JB and Maserejian NN. Associations between Vitamin C Intake and Severity of Lower Urinary Tract Symptoms by Supplemental or Dietary Intake. *BJU Int.* 2015;115(1):134–142.

23. Dallosso H. Nutrient composition of the diet and the development of overactive bladder: A longitudinal study in women. *Neurourol Urodyn.* 2004;15:93–96.

24. Digesu GA, Verdi E, Cardozo L, Olivieri L, Khullar V and Colli E. Phase IIb, multicenter, double-blind, randomized, placebo-controlled, parallel-group study to determine effects of elocalcitol in women with overactive bladder and idiopathic detrusor overactivity. *Urology.* 2012;80:48–54.

25. Kajiwara M and Mutaguchi K. Clinical efficacy and tolerability of gosha-jinki-gan, Japanese traditional herbal medicine, in females with overactive bladder. *Hinyokika Kiyo.* 2008;54:95–99.

26. Ogushi T, Takahashi S. Effect of Chinese herbal medicine on overactive bladder. *Hinyokika Kiyo.* 2007;53:857–862.

27. Noguchi M, Kakuma T and Tomiyasu K. Effect of an extract of Ganoderma lucidum in men with lower urinary tract symptoms: a double-blind placebo- controlled randomized and dose-ranging study. *Asian J Androl.* 2008;10:651–658.

28. Nishimura M, Ohkawara T, Sato H, Takeda H and Nishihira J. Pumpkin Seed Oil Extracted From Cucurbita maxima Improves Urinary Disorder in Human Overactive Bladder. *J Tradit Complement Med.* 2014;4:72–74.

29. Herati AS, Shorter B, Tai J, Lesser M and Moldwin RM. Differences in food sensitivities between female interstitial cystitis/painful bladder syndrome (IC/PBS) and chronic prostatitis/chronic pelvic pain syndrome (CP/CPPS) patients. *J Urol.* 2009;181:22.

30. Kiecolt-Glaser JK, Belury MA, Andridge R, Malarkey WB and Glaser R. Omega-3 supplementation lowers inflammation and anxiety in medical students: A randomized controlled trial. *Brain Behav Immun.* 2011;25:1725–1734.

31. Rogan EG. The natural chemopreventive compound indole-3-carbinol: State of the science, *In Vivo* 2006;20(2):221–228.

32. Rugendorff EW, Weidner W, Ebeling L and Buck AC. Results of treatment with pollen extract (Cernilton N) in chronic prostatitis and prostatodynia. *Br J Urol.* 1993;71:433–438.

33. Carani C, Salvioli V, Scuteri A, *et al.* Urological and sexual evaluation of treatment of benign prostatic disease using Pygeum africanum at high doses. *Arch Ital Urol Nefrol Androl.* 1991;63:341–345.

34. Cai T, Mazzoli S, Bechi A, *et al.* Serenoa repens associated with Urtica dioica (ProstaMEV®) and curcumin and quercitin (FlogMEV®) extracts are able to improve the efficacy of prulifloxacin in bacterial prostatitis patients: results from a prospective randomised study. *Int J Antimicrob Agents.* 2009;33:549–553.

35. Yoon BI, Ha US, Sohn DW, *et al.* Anti-inflammatory and antimicrobial effects of nanocatechin in a chronic bacterial prostatitis rat model. *J Infect Chemother.* 2011;17:189–194.

36. Pitman MS, Cheetham PJ, Hruby GW and Katz AE. Vitamin D deficiency in the urological population: A single center analysis. *J Urol.* 2011;186:1395–1399.

37. Gómez Y, Arocha F, Espinoza F, Fernández D, Vásquez A and Granadillo V. Zinc levels in prostatic fluid of patients with prostate pathologies. *Investigacion clinica.* 2007;48:287–294.

38. Goodarzi D, Cyrus A, Baghinia MR, Kazemifar AM and Shirincar M. The efficacy of zinc for treatment of chronic prostatitis. *Acta medica Indonesiana.* 2013;45:259–264.

39. Liu L, Yang J and Lu F. Urethral dysbacteriosis as an underlying, primary cause of chronic prostatitis: Potential implications for probiotic therapy. *Medical Hypotheses.* 2009;73:741–743.

40. Vicari E, La Vignera S, Castiglione R, Condorelli Ra, Vicari LO and Calogero AE. Chronic bacterial prostatitis and irritable bowel syndrome: effectiveness of treatment with rifaximin followed by the probiotic VSL#3. *Asian J Androl.* 2014:735–739.

41. Teichman JM. Potassium sensitivity testing in the diagnosis and treatment of interstitial cystitis. *Infect Urol.* 2003;16:87–94.

42. Bologna RA, Gomelsky A, Lukban JC, Tu LM, Holzberg AS and Whitmore KE. The efficacy of calcium glycerophosphate in the prevention of food-related flares in interstitial cystitis. *Urology.* 2001;57:119–120.

43. Erickson DR, Morgan KC, Ordille S, Keay SK and Xie SX. Nonbladder related symptoms in patients with interstitial cystitis. *J Urol.* 2001;166:557–561; discussion 561–562.

44. Whitmore KE. Complementary and alternative therapies as treatment approaches for interstitial cystitis. *Rev Urol.* 2002;4 Suppl 1:S28–35.

45. DiPasquale R. Effective use of herbal medicine in urinary tract infections. *J Diet Suppl.* 2008;5:219–228.

46. *Materia Medica: Equisetum arvense*, 547(Healing Arts Press 2003).

47. Smith SD, Wheeler MA, Foster Jr. HE and Weiss RM. Improvement in Interstitial Cystitis Symptom Scores During Treatment With Oral L-Arginine. *J Urol.* 1997;158:703–708.

48. Cartledge JJ, Davies AM and Eardley I. A randomized double-blind placebo-controlled crossover trial of the efficacy of l-arginine in the treatment of interstitial cystitis. *BJU Int.* 2000;85:421–426.

49. Korting GE, Smith SD, Wheeler MA, Weiss RM and Foster Jr. He. A randomized double-blind trial of oral L-arginine for treatment of interstitial cystitis. *J Urol.* 1998;161:558–565.

50. Katske F, Shoskes DA, Sender M, Poliakin R, Gagliano K and Rajfer J. Treatment of interstitial cystitis with a quercetin supplement. *Tech Urol.* 2001;7:44–46.

51. Kurabayashi H, Kubota K, Kawada E, Tamura K, Tamura J and Shirakura T. Complete cure of urinary and faecal incontinence after intravenous vitamin B12 therapy in a patient with post-gastrectomy megaloblastic anaemia. *J Intern Med.* 1992;231:313–315.

52. Dursun M, Otunctemur A, Ozbek E, Sahin S, Besiroglu H and Koklu I. Stress urinary incontinence and visceral adipose index: a new risk parameter. *Int Urol Nephrol.* 2014:1–4.

53. Subak LL, Wing R, West DS, *et al.* Weight loss to treat urinary incontinence in overweight and obese women. *N Engl J Med.* 2009;360:481–490.

54. Prevalence and risk factors for urinary incontinence in women with type 2 diabetes and impaired fasting glucose: Findings from the National Health and Nutrition Examination Survey (NHANES) 2001–2002, Diabetes Care (2006).

55. Suzuki S, Platz EA, Kawachi I, Willett WC and Giovannucci E. Intakes of energy and macronutrients and the risk of benign prostatic hyperplasia. *Am J Clin Nutr.* 2002;75:689–697.

56. Kappas A, Anderson KE, Conney AH, Pantuck EJ, Fishman J and Bradlow HL. Nutrition-endocrine interactions: induction of reciprocal changes in the delta 4-5 alpha-reduction of testosterone and the cytochrome P-450-dependent oxidation of estradiol by dietary macronutrients in man. *Proc Natl Acad Sci USA.* 1983;80: 7646–7649.

57. Troisi RJ, Weiss ST, Parker DR, Sparrow D, Young JB and Landsberg L. Relation of obesity and diet to sympathetic nervous system activity. *Hypertension.* 1991;17:669–677.

58. Parsons JK and Kashefi C. Physical Activity, Benign Prostatic Hyperplasia, and Lower Urinary Tract Symptoms. *Eur Urol.* 2008;53:1228–1235.

59. Kramer G and Marberger M. Could inflammation be a key component in the progression of benign prostatic hyperplasia? *Curr Opin Urol.* 2006;16:25–29.

60. Christudoss P, Selvakumar R, Fleming JJ and Gopalakrishnan G. Zinc status of patients with benign prostatic hyperplasia and prostate carcinoma. *Indian J Urol.* 2011;27.

61. Om AS and Chung KW. Dietary zinc deficiency alters 5 alpha-reduction and aromatization of testosterone and androgen and estrogen receptors in rat liver. *J Nutr.* 1996;126:842–848.

62. Login IS, Thorner MO and MacLeod RM. Zinc may have a physiological role in regulating pituitary prolactin secretion. *Neuroendocrinology.* 1983;37:317–320.

63. Fahim M, Fahim Z, Der R and Harman J. Zinc treatment for reduction of hyperplasia of prostate. *Federation Proceedings.* 1976;35:361.

64. Kristal AR, Arnold KB, Schenk JM, *et al.* Dietary patterns, supplement use, and the risk of symptomatic benign prostatic hyperplasia: results from the prostate cancer prevention trial. *Am J Epidemiol.* 2008;167:925–934.

65. Colli E, Rigatti P, Montorsi F, *et al.* BXL628, a novel vitamin d3 analog arrests prostate growth in patients with benign prostatic hyperplasia: A randomized clinical trial. *Eur Urol.* 2006;49:82–86.

66. Shifren JL, Monz BU, Russo PA, Segreti A and Johannes CB. Sexual problems and distress in United States women: prevalence and correlates. *Obstet Gynecol.* 2008;112:970–978.

67. Graziottin A. Libido: the biologic scenario. *Maturitas.* 2000;34, Supple:S9–S16.

68. Panjari M and Davis SR. DHEA therapy for women: effect on sexual function and wellbeing. *Hum Reprod Update* 2007;13 239–248.

69. Davis SD, Davison S and Donath S and Bell R. CIrculating androgen levels and self-reported sexual function in women. *JAMA.* 2005;294:91–96.

70. Graziotttin A and Leiblum SR. Biological and psychosocial pathophysiology of female sexual dysfunction during the menopausal transition. *J Sex Med.* 2005;2 Suppl 3:133–145.

71. Labrie F, Archer DF, Bouchard C, *et al.* Intravaginal dehydroepiandrosterone (prasterone), a highly efficient treatment of dyspareunia. *Climacteric.* 2011;14(2):282–288.

72. Ito TY, Polan ML, Whipple B and Trant AS. The enhancement of female sexual function with ArginMax, a nutritional supplement, among women differing in menopausal status. *J Sex Marital Ther.* 2006;32:369–378.

73. Mucci M, Carraro C, Mancino P, *et al.* Soy isoflavones, lactobacilli, Magnolia bark extract, vitamin D3 and calcium. Controlled clinical study in menopause. *Minerva Ginecol.* 2006;58:323–334.

74. Errichi S, Bottari A, Belcaro G, *et al.* Supplementation with Pycnogenol(R) improves signs and symptoms of menopausal transition. *Panminerva Med.* 2011;53:65–70.

75. Dording CM, Fisher L, Papakostas G, *et al.* A double-blind, randomized, pilot dose-finding study of maca root (L. Meyenii) for the management of SSRI-induced sexual dysfunction. *CNS Neurosci Ther.* 2008;14:182–191.

76. Ferguson DM, Singh GS, Stedile CP, Alexander JS, Weihmiller MK and Crosby MG. Randomized, placebo-controlled, double blind,

crossover design trial of the efficacy and safety of zestra for women in women with and without female sexual arousal disorder. *J Sex Marital Ther.* 2003;29:33–44.

77. Montorsi P, Montorsi F and Schulman CC. Is Erectile Dysfunction the "Tip of the Iceberg" of a Systemic Vascular Disorder? *Eur Urol.* 2003;44:352–354.

78. Vlachopoulos C, Ioakeimidis N, Terentes-Printzios D and Stefanadis C. The triad: erectile dysfunction–endothelial dysfunction–cardio-vascular disease. *Curr Pharm Des.* 2008;14:3700–3714.

79. Neuzillet Y, Hupertan V, Cour F, Botto H and Lebret T. A random-ized, double-blind, crossover, placebo-controlled comparative clinical trial of arginine aspartate plus adenosine monophosphate for the intermittent treatment of male erectile dysfunction. *Andrology.* 2013;1:223–228.

80. Lebret T, Hervé J-M, Gorny P, Worcel M and Botto H. Efficacy and Safety of a Novel Combination of L-Arginine Glutamate and Yohimbine Hydrochloride: A New Oral Therapy for Erectile Dysfunction. *Eur Urol.* 2002;41:608–613.

81. Paroni R, Barassi A, Ciociola F, *et al.* Asymmetric dimethylarginine (ADMA), symmetric dimethylarginine (SDMA) and L-arginine in patients with arteriogenic and non-arteriogenic erectile dysfunc-tion. *Int J Androl.* 2012;35:660–667.

82. Therapeutic use of citrulline in cardiovascular disease, Cardio-vascular Drug Reviews (2006).

83. Shindel AW, Xin ZC, Lin G, *et al.* Erectogenic and neurotrophic effects of icariin, a purified extract of horny goat weed (Epimedium spp.) *in vitro* and *in vivo. J Sex Med.* 2010;7:1518–1528.

84. Forest CP, Padma-Nathan H and Liker HR. Efficacy and safety of pomegranate juice on improvement of erectile dysfunction in male patients with mild to moderate erectile dysfunction:a randomized, placebo-controlled, double-blind, crossover study. *Int J Impot Res.* 2007;19(6):564–567.

85. Reiter WJ, Pycha A, Schatzl G, *et al.* Dehydroepiandrosterone in the treatment of erectile dysfunction: a prospective, double-blind, randomized, placebo-controlled study. *Urology.* 1999;53(3):590–594.

86. Riley AJ, Riley EJ and Brown P. Biological aspects of sexual desire in women. *J Sex Marital Ther.* 1986;1:35–42.

87. Ettala OO, Syvänen KT, Korhonen PE, *et al.* High-intensity physi-cal activity, stable relationship, and high education level associate with decreasing risk of erectile dysfunction in 1,000 apparently

healthy cardiovascular risk subjects. *J Sex Med.* 2014;11(9): 2277–2284.

88. Romeo JH, Seftel AD, Madhun ZT and Aron DC. Sexual function in men with diabetes type 2: association with glycemic control. *J Urol.* 2000;163:788–791.

89. Esposito K, Ciotola M, Giugliano F, Schisano B, Autorino R, Iuliano S, Vietri MT, Cioffi M, De Sio M and Giugliano D. Mediterranean diet improves sexual function in women with the metabolic syndrome. *Int J Impot Res.* 2007;19(5): 486–491.

90. Wessells H, Penson DF, Cleary P, *et al.* Effect of intensive glycemic therapy on erectile function in men with type 1 diabetes. *J Urol.* 2011;185:1828–1834.

91. Nascimento ER, Maia ACO, Pereira V, Soares-Filho G, Nardi AE and Silva AC. Sexual dysfunction and cardiovascular diseases: a systematic review of prevalence. *Clinics (São Paulo, Brazil).* 2013;68:1462–1468.

92. Liu TC, Lin CH, Huang CY, Ivy JL and Kuo CH. Effect of acute DHEA administration on free testosterone in middle-aged and young men following high-intensity interval training. *Eur J Appl Physiol.* 2013;113:1783–1792.

93. Jedrzejuk D, Medras M, Milewicz A and Demissie M. Dehydroepiandrosterone replacement in healthy men with age-related decline of DHEA-S: effects on fat distribution, insulin sensitivity and lipid metabolism. *Aging Male.* 2003;6(3):151–156.

94. Tambi MIBM, Imran MK and Henkel RR. Standardised water-soluble extract of Eurycoma longifolia, Tongkat ali, as testosterone booster for managing men with late-onset hypogonadism? *Andrologia.* 2012;44:226–230.

95. Gonzales GF, Córdova A, Vega K, *et al.* Effect of Lepidium meyenii (MACA) on sexual desire and its absent relationship with serum testosterone levels in adult healthy men. *Andrologia.* 2002;34: 367–372.

96. Gupta A, Mahdi AA, Shukla KK, *et al.* Efficacy of Withania somnifera on seminal plasma metabolites of infertile males: A proton NMR study at 800 MHz. *J Ethnopharmacol.* 2013;149:208–214.

97. Ahmad MK, Mahdi AA, Shukla KK, Islam N, Jaiswar SP and Ahmad S. Effect of Mucuna pruriens on semen profile and biochemical parameters in seminal plasma of infertile men. *Fertil Steril.* 2008;90:627–635.

98. *Pharmacology and modes of action of extracts of Palmetto fruits (Sabal Fructus), stinging nettle roots (Urticae Radix) and pumpkin seed (Cucurbitae Peponis Semen) in the treatment of benign prostatic hyperplasia*, 55–57(1995).

99. Sellandi T, Thakar A and Baghel M. Clinical study of *Tribulus terrestris* Linn. in Oligozoospermia: A double blind study. *AYU* 2012;33(3):356–364.

100. Qureshi A, Naughton DP and Petroczi A. A systematic review on the herbal extract tribulus terrestris and the roots of its putative aphrodisiac and performance enhancing effect. *J Diet Suppl.* 2014;11:64–79.

101. Netter A, Hartoma R and Nahoul K. Effect of zinc administration on plasma testosterone, dihydrotestosterone, and sperm count. *Arch Androl.* 1981;7:69–73.

102. Vona-Davis L and Rose DP. The obesity-inflammation-eicosanoid axis in breast cancer. *J Mammary Gland Biol Neoplasia.* 2013;18: 291–307.

103. Davies G, Martin L-A, Sacks N and Dowsett M. Cyclooxygenase-2 (COX-2), aromatase and breast cancer: a possible role for COX-2 inhibitors in breast cancer chemoprevention. *Ann Oncol.* 2002;13: 669–678.

104. Meeker JD, Ryan L, Barr DB and Hauser R. Exposure to nonpersistent insecticides and male reproductive hormones. *Epidemiology (Cambridge, Mass.).* 2006;17:61–68.

105. Zawatski W and Lee MM. Male pubertal development: Are endocrine-disrupting compounds shifting the norms? *J Endocrinol.* 2013;218(2):R1–R12.

106. Thoreux-Manlay A, Vélez de la Calle JF, Olivier MF, Soufir JC, Masse R and Pinon-Lataillade G. Impairment of testicular endocrine function after lead intoxication in the adult rat. *Toxicology.* 1995;100:101–109.

107. Shah PJ, Williams G and Green NA. Idiopathic hypercalciuria: its control with unprocessed bran. *Br J Urol.* 1980;52:426–429.

108. Zechner O, Latal D, Pflüger H and Scheiber V. Nutritional risk factors in urinary stone disease. *J Urol.* 1981;125:51–54.

109. Taylor EN, Curhan GC. Fructose consumption and the risk of kidney stones. *Kidney International.* 2008;73:207–212.

110. Lemann J, Piering WF, Lennon EJ, Kelly OA and Brock J. Possible Role of Carbohydrate-Induced Calciuria in Calcium Oxalate Kidney-Stone Formation. *N Engl J Med.* 1969;280:232–237.

111. Nouvenne A, Meschi T, Prati B, *et al*. Effects of a low-salt diet on idiopathic hypercalciuria in calcium-oxalate stone formers: A 3-mo randomized controlled trial. *Am J Clin Nutr.* 2010;91: 565–570.

112. Borghi L, Meschi T, Amato F, Briganti A, Novarini A and Giannini A. Urinary volume, water and recurrences in idiopathic calcium nephrolithiasis: A 5-year randomized prospective study. *J Urol.* 1996;155:839–843.

113. Prien E and Gershoff S. Magnesium oxide-pyridoxine therapy for recurrent calcium oxalate calculi. *J Urol.* 1974;112:509–512.

114. Idiopathic hypocitraturic calcium-oxalate nephrolithiasis successfully treated with potassium citrate, Annals of Internal Medicine (1986).

115. Liebman M and Chai W. Effect of dietary calcium on urinary oxalate excretion after oxalate loads. *Am J Clin Nutr.* 1997;65: 1453–1459.

116. Tang J, McFann KK and Chonchol MB. Association between serum 25-hydroxyvitamin D and nephrolithiasis: the National Health and Nutrition Examination Survey III, 1988-94. *Nephrol Dial Transplant.* 2012;27:4385–4389.

117. Nakagawa T, Hu H, Zharikov S, *et al*. A causal role for uric acid in fructose-induced metabolic syndrome. *Am J Physiol Renal Physiol.* 2006;290:F625–F631.

118. Kumar V, Sinha AK, Makkar HPS and Becker K. Dietary roles of phytate and phytase in human nutrition: a review. *Food Chem.* 2010;120:945–959.

119. Coe F, Moran E and Kavalich A. The contribution of dietary purine over-consumption to hyperpuricosuria in calcium oxalate stone formers. *J Chronic Dis.* 1976;29:793–300.

120. Siener R and Hesse A. The effect of a vegetarian and different omnivorous diets on urinary risk factors for uric acid stone formation. *Eur J Nutr.* 2003;42:332–337.

121. Kessler T, Jansen B and Hesse A. Effect of blackcurrant-, cranberry- and plum juice consumption on risk factors associated with kidney stone formation. *Eur J Clin Nutr.* 2002;56:1020–1023.

122. Massey LK, Liebman M and Kynast-Gales SA. Ascorbate increases human oxaluria and kidney stone risk. Paper presented at: The Journal of nutrition, 2005.

123. Moyad MA, Combs MA, Crowley DC, *et al*. Vitamin C with metabolites reduce oxalate levels compared to ascorbic acid: a preliminary and novel clinical urologic finding. *Urol Nurs.* 2009;29:95–102.

124. Scott R, Cunningham C, McLelland A, Fell GS, Fitzgerald-Finch OP and McKellar N. The importance of cadmium as a factor in calcified upper urinary tract stone disease — a prospective 7-year study. *Br J Urol.* 1982;54:584–589.

125. Alagiri M, Chottiner S, Ratner V, Slade D and Hanno PM. Interstitial cystitis: Unexplained associations with other chronic disease and pain syndromes. *Urology.* 1997;49:52–57.

126. Ohman L, Tornblom H and Simren M. Crosstalk at the mucosal border: importance of the gut microenvironment in IBS. *Nat Rev Gastroenterol Hepatol.* 2015;12(1):36–49.

127. Franco I. The central nervous system and its role in bowel and bladder control. *Curr Urol Rep.* 2011;12:153–157.

128. Coyne KS, Cash B, Kopp Z, *et al*. The prevalence of chronic constipation and faecal incontinence among men and women with symptoms of overactive bladder. *BJU Int.* 2011;107:254–261.

129. Pitkala K, Strandberg T and Finne-Soveri U. Fermented cereal with specific bifidobacteria normalizes bowel movements in elderly nursing home residents. A randomized, controlled trial. *J Nutr Health Aging.* 2007;11:305–311.

130. Gordon D, Groutz A, Ascher-Landsberg J, Lessing JB, David MP and Razz O. Double-blind, placebo-controlled study of magnesium hydroxide for treatment of sensory urgency and detrusor instability: preliminary results. *Br J Obstet Gynaecol.* 1998;105(6):667–669.

Chapter 5

Functional Nutrition for Pelvic Health

Jessica Drummond

The Integrative Women's Health Institute, Houston, Texas

Functional nutrition refers to the practice of nourishing the body with important macronutrients and micronutrients to carry out important chemical activities. This practice has had much success in athletic populations to decrease the incidence of pain in both males and females. Clinically, the use of functional nutrition can have important implications in treating urological disorders such as urinary incontinence, painful bladder symptoms (PBS), and pelvic pain. This branch of medicine is used to discover the root cause(s) of these disorders being experienced by the patient. By changing their nutritional behaviors patients can reduce the degree of the pain. This chapter will address different foods and the important nutrients that can be effective in treating urological diseases.

Introduction

For women and men who struggle with chronic pelvic pain (CPP), fecal and urinary incontinence, painful bladder symptoms (PBS), sexual pain, and loss of sexual desire, it is the perspective of practitioners of functional nutrition that it is essential to get to the root cause of the pain or functional impairment. Many symptoms can be the result of a single root cause, and different root causes can manifest as the same clinical symptom.

One of the best examples of the same underlying condition manifesting in many ways is celiac disease.[1] About half of all adults diagnosed with celiac disease will present with atypical or non-GI findings. In the realm of pelvic health concerns these can include chronic fatigue, fibromyalgia-like complaints, abdominal pain, joint pain-inflammation, constipation and/or diarrhea, bloating and distention, delayed puberty and early menopause. Additionally, about 8% of patients presenting at a peripheral neuropathy center for evaluation were found to have celiac disease.[2] Alternatively a woman with abdominal or pelvic pain, may not have underlying celiac disease. She could have endometriosis, ovarian cysts, pelvic floor muscle dysfunction, uterine fibroids, or other causes of pelvic pain.[3]

The pelvis is a unique bowl within the body that is home to multiple biological systems. When any one of these systems is not functioning optimally, the others can be impacted. In this chapter, we will examine the impacts that nutrition can have on a multitude of pelvic organ impairments, and it's important to note that many of them cross biological systems.

For example, a woman with pelvic pain could have a combination of pelvic floor muscle spasm, the psychological risk factor of a history of sexual abuse, an ovarian cyst due to a new onset of polycystic ovarian syndrome (PCOS), and may be continuing to eat a diet that is high in sugar and other inflammatory foods which will have hormonal impacts on her PCOS and will increase her levels of inflammatory cytokines.

Thus, in this chapter, we will focus on biological and psychological system optimization, nourishment if you will, to discuss within each system how a variety of symptoms in the pelvic region can manifest when those systems are not functioning optimally.

The Immune System and the Impact of Chronic Inflammation on Pelvic Health

It is increasingly understood via the biopsychosocial model of pain that the perception and response to pain combine biological changes, psychological influence, and sociocultural background and surroundings. Thus, the pain response is highly variable across people and at different times even for the same initial trigger. "Pain is widely regarded as a complex phenomenon with inputs from biological nociceptive and hypothalamic-pituitary-adrenal axis activity, as well as psychosocial and socio-economic factors such as emotional disposition, cognition and attention, functional and subjective disability, and system-of-care issues".[4] Pain is not a one-to-one relationship with inflammation, however, inflammation continues to play a role as one aspect of the biological contribution to pain.

From a nutrition perspective, any foods or chronic stressors that trigger the immune system to release inflammatory cytokines can contribute to chronic pain or other pelvic health issues that have been associated with elevated markers of inflammation. Finding which foods will do so in each person takes an individualized approach. The best method to use as a nutritionist, is to use a specific elimination diet. Exactly how to implement an elimination diet to assess an individual patient's triggers is detailed below.

When it comes to pelvic pain conditions including endometriosis, vulvodynia, and PBS, the complex relationship between the brain and the digestive and immune systems coordinates the release of inflammatory cytokines, which can impact pain perception and intensity. It is known in animal models that inflammatory cytokines influence and stimulate the HPA axis and the serotonin and dopamine pathways.[5] Now the human model of depression is being used to look at the influence of the immune system via inflammation on the nervous system. There are nearly 200 published studies looking at the relationship between inflammation and depression. This relationship could be even more important in women because women appear to be disproportionately affected by several factors that elevate inflammation, including prior depression, somatic symptomatology, interpersonal stressors, childhood adversity, obesity, and physical inactivity.[6] Relationship distress and obesity, both of which elevate depression risk, are more strongly linked to inflammation for women than for men.

Stressors (physical, emotional, or spiritual) stimulate the hypothalamic–pituitary–adrenal axis, triggering the release of hormones that stimulate the immune system and the release of inflammatory cytokines. Stressors to the intestinal mucosa can also trigger this same immune response (discussed in more detail later in this chapter). Encouraging a vicious cycle, the inflammatory cytokines can act on the brain as stressors maintaining the inflammation and pain signaling.

In a number of conditions associated with pelvic pain, elevated inflammatory markers have been found. Several cytokines including interleukin (IL)-1, 6, 8, 10, tumor necrosis factor (TNF)-α, and vascular endothelial growth factor (VEGF) were found to be increased in the peritoneal fluid of women with endometriosis.[7] Endometriotic lesions have been found to produce IL-17A and the removal of the lesions via laparoscopic surgery leads to the significant reduction in the systemic levels of IL-17A.[8] There is likely an important role of IL-17A in promoting angiogenesis and a proinflammatory environment in the peritoneal cavity for the establishment and maintenance of endometriosis lesions.

Using nutrition strategies, what can be done to reduce inflammation in the pelvic region?

Foods and herbs including green tea, turmeric, white willow bark, ginger, omega-3 essential fatty acids, and boswella in athletic populations have been found to impact the inflammatory cascade by inhibiting enzymatic reactions.[9] Specifically for women with dysmenorrhea, 95 women in a double-blind crossover study took one omega-3 capsule for three months, and decreased the intensity of their dysmenorrhea and reduced the need for ibuprofen rescue doses.[10] Thymus vulgaris essential oil, 2% has similar pain reducing effects for women with primary dysmenorrhea.[11] However, the safety of ingesting essential oils, especially on the health of the gut microbiota is still up for debate.

Some specific foods have been studied for their anti-inflammatory activity. Spices such as cinnamon, cloves, and oregano were all found to have anti-inflammatory activity, oregano being the most active.[12] Foods such as lime zest, English breakfast tea, onion, sweet potato, honey-brown mushroom, button mushroom, oyster mushroom, raw oyster mushrooms, shiitake mushrooms, and enoki mushrooms also have demonstrated anti-inflammatory properties. All mushrooms were found to have some benefit, and the onion, sweet potato, raw oyster mushrooms, shiitake mushrooms, and enoki mushrooms were found to be the most powerful.

Some anti-inflammatory supplements have been studied specifically in pelvic pain. In a randomized, controlled clinical trial, men with pelvic pain were given a placebo for 12 weeks, then a supplement containing pollen extracts (Cernitin GBX and Cernitin T60) for 12 weeks.[13] Improvements were seen the NIH-Chronic Prostatitis Symptoms Index (NIH-CPSI) scores, NIH-CPSI pain domain scores and NIH-CPSI quality of life domain scores. Supplemental quercetin, an antioxidant, has also been studied in men with pelvic pain. In a double-blind placebo controlled trial, a one month course of placebo or quercitin (500 mg twice daily) was given to the subjects.[14] NIH-CPSI scores improved from 20.2 to 18.8 in the placebo group and reduced from 21.0 to 13.1 ($p <$ 0.05) in those receiving the quercitin. Seventeen additional patients were given Prosta-Q, a supplement containing quercitin, plus digestive enzymes bromelain and papain to promote intestinal absorption. Only 20% of the placebo group had greater than 25% improvement vs. 82% of those taking Prosta-Q had a greater than 25% improvement in symptoms. In animal data, the antioxidant lycopene has been found to enhance the effectiveness of ciprofloxacin in the treatment of chronic bacterial prostatitis.[15]

In women, eating an inflammatory, high glycemic diet has been shown to increase bacterial vaginosis acquisition and persistence.[16] In mouse models, the powerful antioxidant vitamin C has been shown to significantly reduce the volumes and weights of endometriotic cysts.[17] Those mice who received the highest vitamin C dose had the lowest cyst volume.

Hydration status has demonstrated effect on the functioning of the epithelium. While research has not been done on hydration and the intestinal epithelium, it is well known that both the epithelium and the intestinal epithelium serve as external and internal "skin" or protective semipermeable barrier layers. Hydration status even affects the inflammatory signaling at the genetic level of epidermal wound healing, and is likely to have a similar effect on the healing of the intestinal mucosal barrier.

The importance of healthy intestinal barrier function

In 2012, Dr. Fasano published an important paper linking the loss of healthy intestinal barrier function to a protein in gluten containing foods.[18] Other proteins, such as claudin-2 up regulation also contribute to increased permeability in intestinal barrier function. Stress, non-steroidal anti-inflammatory drugs, and even intense exercise with restricted fluid intake contribute to the breakdown of healthy intestinal barrier function. Once the barrier function is compromised, common foods can trigger an inflammatory response from the immune system. Determining which foods are doing so in a specific individual can be determined by a systematic elimination diet protocol.

In pelvic pain, a few studies have identified some common food triggers across patients. In one Italian study, 330 women with endometriosis confirmed by ultrasound, MRI, and laparoscopy, excluding women with confirmed celiac disease, were put on a gluten free diet for 12 months.[19] They were educated to be completely gluten free including foods, medications, vitamins, skincare, and cosmetics. Of the 207 women who completed the study, 156 (75%) reported significant improvement in symptoms,

51 (25%) reported no change in symptoms. All 207 women reported improvements in physical functioning, general health perception, vitality, social functioning, and mental health. Importantly, this study has significant limitations since 123 women (nearly 40% of the subjects) withdrew from the study or refused to participate.

Several case studies have been published of women with endometriosis using dietary strategies in either failed medical cases or in addition to standard medical treatment using elimination diets to reduce pain and restore fertility.[20] Interestingly, in each case the foods found to trigger symptoms were highly variable, primarily sugar and grains in one case, and sugar, milk, yeast, nightshade vegetables, and eggs in another case.

Cases of women with a combination of pelvic symptoms including endometriosis, dysmenorrhea, uterine polyps, abnormal bleeding, and uterine leiomyomas have also been published looking at the impact of nutrition on symptoms.[21] In these cases, high levels of intake of dietary soy, once removed, resulted in dramatic improvements in symptoms and normalization of fertility.

The elimination diet as a diagnostic tool for personalizing nutrition recommendations in patients with pelvic pain, low libido, constipation, or continence issues

Based on a review of the pelvic pain, infertility and nutrition literature, our Integrative Women's Health Institute, has determined a specific elimination diet protocol for determining possible food triggers for pain, fatigue, and low libido in our patients with pelvic health conditions.[22] For at least three weeks, gluten, beef, eggs, sugar, artificial sweeteners, dairy, nightshade vegetables, citrus fruits, soy, peanuts, corn, coffee, baker's yeast, and onions are eliminated from the diet. Patients are encouraged to eat an anti-inflammatory Mediterranean style diet including organic poultry, wild fish, non-nightshade vegetables and root vegetables, nuts and seeds (except for peanuts which are legumes), olive oil, coconut oil, and avocado since it is known that a diet high in vegetables and omega-3 fats reduces risk of endometriosis.[23] In some individual cases where bloating is a symptom, all legumes and grains are also temporarily eliminated.

Once these potential nutritional triggers have been eliminated for three weeks, if there is noticeable symptom improvement, we will recommend adding each food back into the diet for four days, 2–3 servings per day, with journaling of symptoms. If no symptoms are triggered, then the food is safe to continue in the diet. If pain, skin breakouts, itching, digestive issues, headaches, menstrual changes, mood changes, sleep difficulty, brain fog, heart rate or rhythm changes, or weight gain occur, then the food is eliminated for at least six months before challenging again. When the symptoms resolve from the challenge, the next food challenge is initiated.

We have found clinically that this approach is superior to simply removing the foods that have been found to most commonly trigger urologic and pelvic pain in men and women by patient report, foods such as spicy foods, coffee, tea and other caffeine sources, citrus fruits, vinegar, and alcoholic beverages. However, in patients with urologic complaints such as painful bladder syndrome or interstitial cystitis (IC), adding these common irritants to the more comprehensive elimination protocol is recommended. Without implementing the more individualized systematic elimination diet, foods that do trigger symptoms, such as gluten or dairy which have limited data support, but are clinically relevant to many individuals, may be missed.

The optimal diet will be ineffective if the nutrients are not absorbed

In addition to the health of the intestinal epithelium, the entire digestive process must be functioning effectively in order to optimize health. When we reimagine the old adage, "You are what you eat." as "You are what you absorb." we can consider the role of digestive health as impacting pelvic health.

According to a study presented at the 2013 Institute of Food Technologists Annual Meeting and Food Expo in Chicago, IL, chewing almonds 40 times was the optimal number of chews for maximal absorption of the food. Then, once food enters the stomach, adequate acidity must be present for intrinsic factor to support the absorption of vitamin B12 and for the activation of pepsin for effective breakdown of proteins.[24] In the duodenum, where the pH begins to rise, bile salts mix with triglycerides, and pancreatic enzymes are released. Iron, magnesium, selenium, calcium and other minerals and vitamins are absorbed in the duodenum. In the jejunum many nutrients are absorbed, including calcium, folate, zinc, free fatty acids, many B vitamins, fat soluble vitamins A, D, E and K, vitamin B12, and some water and sodium are absorbed. In the ileum, vitamin C, folate, vitamin D, vitamin K, vitamin B12, magnesium and other minerals, water, and sodium, are absorbed, and bile acids are recycled. In the colon, electrolytes are absorbed along with water, vitamin K, biotin, and short chain fatty acids many of which are produced by the gut microbes. Finally, elimination of waste is the essential completion of the process.

The health of the gut microbiota is essential to digestive function, to the production of nutrients, and to reducing risk of bacterial and yeast infections. Variations in the gut microbiota between patients with and without pelvic visceral hypersensitivity have been found.[25] The intestinal microbiota in irritable bowel syndrome (IBS) patients differs from that in healthy individuals, with a consistent decrease in the Bifidobacterium species population and an increase in the Enterobacter population, plus other studies have found differences including an increased ratio of Firmicutes to Bacteroidetes and a reduction in Lactobacillus species in those with IBS.[25] It may be critical to establish a healthy gut microbiota in early life in order to reduce the risk of later visceral pain. Disruption of the microbiome during early life by administration of vancomycin for postnatal day 4–13 led to visceral hypersensitivity to colorectal distension in adult rats, even though the dysbiosis had resolved.[25] Specific probiotics and probiotic strains have been found to attenuate visceral pain. *L. rhamnosus* ATCC 53103 (Lactobacillus GG; LGG), and a prebiotic mix of galactooligosaccharides and polydextrose expressed significant analgesic effect.[25] The prebiotics to a less extent compared to the probiotic strain LGG. LGG was found to alter the levels of brain neurotransmitters, like serotonin, noradrenaline, and dopamine which are known to be involved in pain modulation. Treatment with live and killed Lactobacillus reuteri prevented the pain response to colorectal distension by decreasing of the dorsal root ganglion single unit activity to distension.[25] A decrease of normal visceral perception and chronic colonic hypersensitivity, elicited by butyrate was also observed after an oral treatment by *L. acidophilus* NCFM.[25] A mixture of eight probiotic bacteria strains (VSL#3) has been shown to have protective effects against development of visceral hypersensitivity and to prevent visceral hypersensitivity induced by inflammation via intracolonic instillation of 4% acetic acid when given prophylactically.[26] Bifidobacterium species particularly, Bifidobacterium infantis 35624 has been shown to be particularly effective at ameliorating visceral hyperalgesia in both stress-induced visceral hypersensitivity and colitis.[26]

It is increasingly understood that it is important to carefully choose specific strains when using probiotic supplements therapeutically. Specific strains have been found to be useful to prevent and treat bacterial vaginosis (BV). Lactobacillus strains (Lactobacillus brevis CD2, *L. salivarius* FV2, and *L. plantarum* FV9), present in Florisia vaginal tablets — a probiotic product for vaginal use — have been selected for properties relating to mucosal colonization, i.e. their ability to adhere at high levels to human epithelial cells and to temporarily colonize the human vagina, for the production of antimicrobial compounds effective towards BV-related microorganisms and for the capacity to inhibit pathogen binding to the cell membrane.[27] Florisia vaginal tablets have been assessed for effectiveness in the treatment of symptomatic bacterial vaginosis in a double-blind placebo-controlled clinical trial. Treatment with the probiotic preparation was 61% effective in eliminating BV and 50% effective in restoring "normal vaginal flora" as determined by Gram stain three weeks after therapy.[27] The efficacy of vaginal probiotic treatment on the recurrence rate of BV has also been evaluated. Lactobacillus supplementation (EcoVag®Vaginal capsules containing L. gasseri Lba EB01-DSM 14869 and L. rhamnosus Lbp PB01-DSM 14870) or probiotic prophylaxis with vaginal capsules containing *L. rhamnosus*, *L. acidophilus*, and *Streptococcus thermophilus* (Probaclac Vaginal) resulted in lower recurrence rates for BV.[27]

Nutritionally, there is time proven value in using probiotic foods to more generally support the health of the gut microbiota and colon until more is known about the optimal supplemental strains to recommend for specific individuals. Homemade sauerkraut, yogurt, kimchi, lacto-fermented vegetables, miso, kefir, and poi are having a culinary resurgence recently in Western cultures. However, fermenting foods has been in use for thousands of years to preserve foods outside of their growing season, and to increase variety in healthy diets when refrigeration was less readily available.

Unfortunately, the Standard Western Diet, which is high in fat, sugar, processed foods and trans fats, and low in probiotics, prebiotics, enzymes, omega-3 fatty acids, and micronutrients can negatively impact the functioning of the digestive process and of the health of the gut microbiota.[28] Whole foods diets rich in a variety of vegetables, high quality proteins, prebiotics and probiotics, omega-3 fatty acid sources and low in processed sugars, fats and carbohydrates promote health in a number of areas including the prevention of cancer, cardiovascular disease, and autoimmune conditions.

Research on Dietary Patterns and Pelvic Health

When it comes to pelvic health conditions research is scarcer, but there are some published studies that do link similar overall healthy nutrition recommendations to improvements in function and reduction of pelvic symptoms.

Regular, moderate red wine consumption (1–2 glasses per day), a key recommendation in the well known, whole food,

Mediterranean Diet, has been associated with improvements in Female Sexual Function Index (FSFI) scores in the domains of sexual desire, lubrication, and overall sexual function. Moderate red wine drinking in men (1–3 times per week) has been correlated with fewer sperm neck abnormalities ($p = 0.01$).[29]

Omega-3 fatty acid consumption may reduce some of the sexual side effects of statin drugs,[30] and omega-3 fatty acid levels may play a role in endometriosis and ovarian cyst risks,[31] however, the data in these conditions is sparse and not yet detailed enough to apply clinically. For erectile dysfunction the data are more clear that erectile dysfunction is a clinical indicator for undiagnosed diabetes and future cardiovascular disease, thus in men with erectile dysfunction clinical nutrition recommendations for reducing diabetes and cardiovascular disease can not only restore sexual function, but can also potentially prove to be lifesaving. For those who are diagnosed with early Type 2 diabetes, a low carbohydrate Mediterranean diet can increase rates of remission and decrease the need for medication. Omega-3 fatty acids and restoring the balance of the omega-6: omega-3 fatty acid ratio may also have positive effects on urologic inflammation.

Mineral deficiencies can also play a role in pelvic health concerns. Men with low or excessive selenium levels may have sperm abnormalities, low sperm motility, and reduced fertility.[32] Low selenium levels can also affect male libido. Foods rich in selenium include Brazil nuts, oysters, liver, tuna, shrimp, sardines, and salmon. Saw palmetto supplementation with the addition of selenium and the antioxidant lycopene performed better to reduce NIH-CPSI scores, pain, PSA levels, and white blood cell counts in subjects with IIIa chronic prostatitis/chronic pelvic pain syndrome (IIIa CP/CPPS). Dietary therapy including vitamin and mineral supplementation, probiotic foods, and fish oil supports improvements in pain and quality of life after surgery for endometriosis stages III and IV.

For women with PCOS, symptoms can include loss of libido, pelvic pain, and dyspareunia. In this syndrome, we can see a number of mechanisms contributing to symptoms, including insulin resistance, mineral deficiencies (especially in chromium which can impact insulin resistance) and an elevated omega-6:omega-3 fatty acid ratio. Dietary recommendations to impact the pain, libido, and fertility symptoms in some women with PCOS are focused on limiting the consumption of sugar and refined carbohydrates, preferring those with lower glycemic index.[33] Additionally, increasing the intake of fish to 12–16 ounces in approximately four servings per week or taking omega-3 fatty acid supplements can be beneficial. Plus, if serum levels are low, taking Vitamin D and chromium supplementation can positively impact symptoms and their underlying causes.

Impact of Nutrition, Hormonal Imbalance and the Detoxification of Estrogen on Pelvic Health

The health of the endocrine and detoxification systems are as important to pelvic health as the health of the digestive, neurologic, and immune systems as discussed above. Endometriosis, ovarian cysts, fibroids, dysmenorrhea, and low libido are all influenced by estrogen dominance. While studies have not been done on using estrogen detoxification strategies on pelvic pain conditions, a model for using nutrients and dietary recommendations to normalize estrogen levels and estrogen to progesterone ratios comes from available literature in breast cancer. In premenopausal women, higher amounts of cruciferous vegetable intake demonstrated a statistically significant association with a decreased risk of breast cancer. Supplemental use of some active components of cruciferous vegetables, 3,3'-diindolylmethane (DIM)[34] and 1-benzyl-indole-3-carbinol are more controversial in the literature, but commonly used in practice to support optimal estrogen metabolism. From a nutrition perspective, using whole cruciferous vegetables is preferable to supplements because in addition to the estrogen metabolizing compounds found within the vegetables are other essential nutrients including minerals, vitamins, and polyphenols. Fermented cruciferous vegetables, such as sauerkraut and kimchi, add supportive probiotics as well.

Low estrogen levels can also be a challenge for women with dyspareunia due to vulvodynia, or thinning and fragile vulvar tissues.

Drinking more caffeinated coffee has been associated with higher sex hormone-binding globulin (SHBG) in post-menopausal women newly diagnosed with diabetes,[35] and with lower estrogen levels in pre-menopausal women.[36] A recent placebo controlled study on using pomegranate oil to alleviate menopause symptoms did not show the increase in estrogen levels of earlier, less rigorous data.[37] But, there was some improvement in symptoms that was non-significantly better than placebo. Flaxseeds have been found to be helpful to enhance immune molecules in breast cancer that are negatively correlated with estrogen levels,[38] but dietary flax does not enhance the effect of estrogen therapy in animal data. Thus, while the data is limited for women with low estrogen, there may be some benefit to adding pomegranate and other foods high in polyphenols, and foods high in fiber and omega-3 fatty acids such as flaxseeds.

Conclusions

The goal of individualized functional nutrition therapy is to supply the body's systems with the micronutrients and macronutrients that it needs to optimally carry out all of its biochemical functions. Optimal functioning of the digestive system is essential to allow for the absorption of a nutrient dense diet and to maintain a healthy immune response. Optimal functioning of the detoxification and endocrine systems are also important to allow for the metabolism of xenobiotics and estrogen. Men and women with pelvic pain and low libido need us to look not just at their diagnosis for clues about nutrition and lifestyle recommendations, but also to how their unique body is able to tolerate the recommendations. Do they have adequate digestive capacity to absorb the food that we are recommending? Do they have adequate liver health and endocrine balance to metabolize the foods and xenobiotics to which they are they are regularly exposed? Finally, as seen with a wider lens, nourishment of the body involves nourishment on all levels, emotional, spiritual and within healthy relationships in addition to the nourishment that can be provided by food, sleep, movement, and exposure to sun and other elements of nature. Our relationships with our patients and our empowerment of our patients to make daily choices in support of nourishing relationships, food choices and lifestyle decisions are the keys to resolving the root causes of each challenging symptom.

References

1. Strauch KA and Cotter VT. Celiac Disease: An Overview and Management for Primary Care Nurse Practitioners. *J Nurse Pract.* 2011;7:588–594.
2. Green PH. The many faces of celiac disease: clinical presentation of celiac disease in the adult population. *Gastroenterology.* 2005;128:S74–S78.
3. Learman LA, Nakagawa S, Gregorich SE, Jackson RA, Jacoby A and Kuppermann M. Success of uterus-preserving treatments for abnormal uterine bleeding, chronic pelvic pain, and symptomatic fibroids: age and bridges to menopause. *Am J Obstet Gynecol.* 2011;204:272. e271–272.e277.
4. Gatchel RJ, McGeary DD, McGeary CA and Lippe B. Interdisciplinary chronic pain management: past, present, and future. *Am Psychol.* 2014;69:119–130.
5. Schedlowski M, Engler H and Grigoleit JS. Endotoxin-induced experimental systemic inflammation in humans: a model to disentangle immune-to-brain communication. *Brain Behav Immun.* 2014;35:1–8.
6. Derry HM, Padin AC, Kuo JL, Hughes S and Kiecolt-Glaser JK. Sex Differences in Depression: Does Inflammation Play a Role? *Curr Psychiatry Rep.* 2015;17:78.
7. Wu MY and Ho HN. The role of cytokines in endometriosis. *Am J Reprod Immunol.* 2003;49:285–296.
8. Ahn SH, Edwards AK, Singh SS, Young SL, Lessey BA and Tayade C. IL-17A Contributes to the Pathogenesis of Endometriosis by Triggering Proinflammatory Cytokines and Angiogenic Growth Factors. *J Immunol.* 2015;195:2591–2600.
9. Maroon JC, Bost JW, Borden MK, Lorenz KM and Ross NA. Natural antiinflammatory agents for pain relief in athletes. *Neurosurg Focus.* 2006;21:E11.

10. Rahbar N, Asgharzadeh N and Ghorbani R. Effect of omega-3 fatty acids on intensity of primary dysmenorrhea. *Int J Gynaecol Obstet.* 2012;117:45–47.
11. Salmalian H, Saghebi R, Moghadamnia AA, *et al.* Comparative effect of thymus vulgaris and ibuprofen on primary dysmenorrhea: A triple-blind clinical study. *Caspian J Intern Med.* 2014;5:82–88.
12. Gunawardena D, Shanmugam K, Low M, *et al.* Determination of anti-inflammatory activities of standardised preparations of plant- and mushroom-based foods. *Eur J Nutr.* 2014;53:335–343.
13. Herati AS and Moldwin RM. Alternative therapies in the management of chronic prostatitis/chronic pelvic pain syndrome. *World J Urol.* 2013;31:761–766.
14. Shoskes DA, Zeitlin SI, Shahed A and Rajfer J. Quercetin in men with category III chronic prostatitis: a preliminary prospective, double-blind, placebo-controlled trial. *Urology.* 1999;54:960–963.
15. Han CH, Yang CH, Sohn DW, Kim SW, Kang SH and Cho YH. Synergistic effect between lycopene and ciprofloxacin on a chronic bacterial prostatitis rat model. *Int J Antimicrob Agents.* 2008;31 (Suppl 1):S102–S107.
16. Thoma ME, Klebanoff MA, Rovner AJ, *et al.* Bacterial vaginosis is associated with variation in dietary indices. *J Nutr.* 2011;141: 1698–1704.
17. Durak Y, Kokcu A, Kefeli M, Bildircin D, Celik H and Alper T. Effect of vitamin C on the growth of experimentally induced endometriotic cysts. *J Obstet Gynaecol Res.* 2013;39:1253–1258.
18. Fasano A. Leaky gut and autoimmune diseases. *Clin Rev Allergy Immunol.* 2012;42:71–78.
19. Marziali M, Venza M, Lazzaro S, Lazzaro A, Micossi C and Stolfi VM. Gluten-free diet: a new strategy for management of painful endometriosis related symptoms? *Minerva Chir.* 2012;67:499–504.
20. Morrison JA, Sullivan J. A novel approach to treating endometriosis: a report on two cases. 1999:225–229.
21. Chandrareddy A, Muneyyirci-Delale O, McFarlane SI and Murad OM. Adverse effects of phytoestrogens on reproductive health: a report of three cases. *Complement Ther Clin Pract.* 2008;14:132–135.
22. Denton C. The elimination/challenge diet. *Minn Med.* 2012;95: 43–44.
23. Parazzini F, Vigano P, Candiani M and Fedele L. Diet and endometriosis risk: a literature review. *Reprod Biomed Online.* 2013;26:323–336.

24. Lipski E. *Digestive Wellness.* McGraw-Hill; 2004.
25. Chichlowski M and Rudolph C. Visceral pain and gastrointestinal microbiome. *J Neurogastroenterol Motil.* 2015;21:172–181.
26. Moloney RD, O'Mahony SM, Dinan TG and Cryan JF. Stress-induced visceral pain: toward animal models of irritable-bowel syndrome and associated comorbidities. *Front Psychiatry.* 2015;6:15.
27. Mastromarino P, Hemalatha R, Barbonetti A, *et al.* Biological control of vaginosis to improve reproductive health. *Indian J Med Res.* 2014;140 Suppl:S91–S97.
28. Brown K, DeCoffe D, Molcan E and Gibson DL. Diet-induced dysbiosis of the intestinal microbiota and the effects on immunity and disease. *Nutrients.* 2012;4:1095–1119.
29. Jurewicz J, Radwan M, Sobala W, *et al.* Lifestyle and semen quality: role of modifiable risk factors. *Syst Biol Reprod Med.* 2014;60: 43–51.
30. Tuccori M, Montagnani S, Mantarro S, *et al.* Neuropsychiatric adverse events associated with statins: epidemiology, pathophysiology, prevention and management. *CNS Drugs.* 2014;28:249–272.
31. Kim TH, Jo S, Park Y, Lee HH, Chung SH and Lee WS. Differences in omega-3 and fatty acid profiles between patients with endometriosis and those with a functional ovarian cyst. *J Obstet Gynaecol.* 2013;33:597–600.
32. Ahsan U, Kamran Z, Raza I, *et al.* Role of selenium in male reproduction — a review. *Anim Reprod Sci.* 2014;146:55–62.
33. Barr S, Reeves S, Sharp K and Jeanes YM. An isocaloric low glycemic index diet improves insulin sensitivity in women with polycystic ovary syndrome. *J Acad Nutr Diet.* 2013;113:1523–1531.
34. Marques M, Laflamme L, Benassou I, Cissokho C, Guillemette B and Gaudreau L. Low levels of 3,3′-diindolylmethane activate estrogen receptor alpha and induce proliferation of breast cancer cells in the absence of estradiol. *BMC Cancer.* 2014;14:524.
35. Goto A, Song Y, Chen BH, Manson JE, Buring JE and Liu S. Coffee and caffeine consumption in relation to sex hormone-binding globulin and risk of type 2 diabetes in postmenopausal women. *Diabetes.* 2011;60:269–275.
36. Kotsopoulos J, Eliassen AH, Missmer SA, Hankinson SE and Tworoger SS. Relationship between caffeine intake and plasma sex hormone concentrations in premenopausal and postmenopausal women. *Cancer.* 2009;115:2765–2774.

37. Auerbach L, Rakus J, Bauer C, *et al.* Pomegranate seed oil in women with menopausal symptoms: a prospective randomized, placebo-controlled, double-blinded trial. *Menopause.* 2012;19:426–432.
38. Abrahamsson A, Morad V, Saarinen NM and Dabrosin C. Estradiol, tamoxifen, and flaxseed alter IL-1beta and IL-1Ra levels in normal human breast tissue *in vivo. J Clin Endocrinol Metab.* 2012;97: E2044–E2054.

Chapter 6

Acupuncture

Jillian Capodice

Assistant Professor, Director of the Integrative Urology and Wellness Program, Department of Urology, Icahn School of Medicine, Mount Sinai Medical Center, New York

Over the past 15 years the use of acupuncture in the clinical setting has advanced and it is now a more widely accepted, safe and effective procedure. Acupuncture is the insertion of fine, sterile needles into the body based on a system of meridians derived from traditional Asian medicine theories. Acupuncture has been proven to be an effective treatment for a variety of indications proven in large multicenter clinical trials. Indications include post-operative pain, post-operative nausea, chemotherapy-induced nausea and vomiting, chronic low back pain, knee osteoarthritis, and migraine headache. In the urologic setting, research and clinical applications of acupuncture for urologic conditions include chronic prostatitis/chronic pelvic pain syndrome, prevention of uncomplicated urinary tract infection (UTI), treatment of lower urinary tract symptoms (LUTS) and as symptom management for a variety of oncologic side effects such as pain, fatigue, and androgen deprivation-induced hot flashes. This chapter will outline the evidence base and highlight the clinical application of acupuncture for numerous urologic conditions.

Recurrent Urinary Tract Infection (rUTI) in Women

rUTI in the lower urinary tract is common among healthy women with normal anatomy and physiology. The incidence rate in women has been shown to be approximately 53,067 cases per 100,000 women in women between the ages of 16 and 35 years old.[1] The recurrence rates of UTI have been shown to range from 27% to 46% over a 12-month period.[2] The pathogenesis of rUTI is thought to be identical to those women with sporadic infection and uropathogens are thought to ascend to the bladder from rectal flora.[3] Other evidence has shown that alteration of normal vaginal flora may be a risk factor for *E. coli* UTI.[4] In pre-menopausal women the most common risk factors for UTI include behavioral risk factors, sexual activity, normal female anatomy (shorter distance between the urethra and the anus) and vitamin D deficiency.[5] In post-menopausal women, the most common risk factors are estrogen deficiency, cystocele, previous history of urogenital surgery, high post-void residual and age-related alterations in vaginal flora.[3,5] Biologic and genetic factors for all women include genetic variability in the IL-8R receptor and family history.[5] The most common prophylactic strategy for women with rUTI includes lifestyle modifications, chronic antibiotic prophylaxis and post-coital prophylaxis.[3] Non-antibiotic prophylaxis strategies include estrogen therapy, cranberry, ascorbic acid, or d-mannose supplementation, probiotics, vaccines, and acupuncture have been investigated.[5,6] A recent meta-analysis suggests that acupuncture may be a useful prophylactic therapy for UTI and two clinical studies performed by the same group of investigators, have demonstrated decreased rUTI rates in women who had received acupuncture.[5–7] In the first study, 67 women were randomized into three groups: true acupuncture, sham acupuncture or no treatment (2:2:1). Acupuncture was administered twice weekly for a total of eight visits over a four-week period. Stainless steel acupuncture needles were inserted, *de qi* (a sensation of soreness or distention that is characteristic for accurate acupuncture needle insertion) was obtained and needles were manipulated with rotation and lifting and thrusting needle techniques. The set of acupuncture points were conception vessel 3 (CV3), urinary bladder 23 and 28 (BL 23, BL28), kidney 3 (KI3), spleen 6 (SP6), liver 2 and liver 3 (LV2, LV3). The clinician performing the procedure was also allowed to choose a combination of additional points (unspecified) for individual patients. For the sham acupuncture procedure, six needles were inserted superficially in non-acupuncture point locations. Superficial needling is one of commonly utilized control groups, however, the exact location of the sham points was not noted in the manuscript. Subjects were followed for six months and repeat urine cultures were obtained. Results demonstrated that there were half as many episodes of uncomplicated UTIs per person in the acupuncture vs. sham vs. no treatment and 85% of patients in the acupuncture group had lower rates of UTI during the six-month follow up vs. 58% of the sham and 36% of the no treatment control group.[7] Side effects in the acupuncture and sham groups were minimal. In the second study, 100 women aged 18–60 were recruited for participation. At baseline, women had to have had three or more episodes of lower urinary tract symptoms (LUTS) during the past year and at least two cases that were diagnosed as acute uncomplicated UTIs. Subjects were randomized 3:1 to acupuncture vs. no treatment. The acupuncture protocol used in this study included only the details of needling and treatment regimen as based on the Standards for Reporting Interventions in Clinical Trials of Acupuncture (STRICTA) characteristics.[8] The needling details included the listing of acupuncture points including: CV3, CV4, BL23, BL28, KI3, SP6, SP9, Stomach 36 (ST36), and LV3 *de qi* was obtained. Treatment frequency was twice weekly for four weeks. The primary outcome was the number of occurrences of acute UTI during the six-month follow up. Results demonstrated that 73% of women in the acupuncture group were free of UTIs during the six-month observation period, as compared with 52% of women in the control group (P = 0.08). The authors also noted that there were 1/3 fewer reported LUTS in the acupuncture group vs. the control group (RR = 0.30; 95% CI = 0.16, 0.58; $P \leq$ 0.01).[9] The most recent meta-analysis of treatment approaches for UTI prophylaxis rates rated them using confidence intervals and a Jadad score (a scale that assigns scores from 0 to 5 based on study characteristics such as randomization and other study quality measures) (Jadad 2, RR 0.48, 95% CI 0.29–0.79). In comparison, vaginal estrogens showed a trend toward preventing rUTI two trials (Jadad 2.5, RR 0.42, 95% CI 0.16–1.10)[7]. While these studies are promising, more studies are needed in order to see if these results are reproducible in larger populations. Moreover, the mechanism for acupuncture in preventing rUTI is not well understood and an additional hypothesis for mechanism of action is improvement of innate immunity.

Interstitial Cystitis (IC) and Bladder Pain Syndrome (PBS)

IC and BPS are part of a symptom complex that includes a variety of patients with LUTS despite sterile urine cultures. Many of these conditions have unknown etiologies. According to the most updated American Urological Association (AUA) guideline, IC and BPS are defined as "an unpleasant sensation (pain, pressure, and discomfort) perceived to be related to the urinary bladder, associated with LUTS of more than six weeks duration, in the absence of infection or other identifiable causes".[10,11] The prevalence of IC/BPS varies widely and patient reported studies have indicated an incidence of about 83,000 male and 1.2 million female cases per year according the National Health Interview Survey (NHIS) and National Health and Nutrition Examination Surveys (NHANES III).[10] The typical course of the condition and comorbidities include diagnosis in the 4th decade or later in life, initial symptoms such as dysuria, frequency or pain with progression to multiple symptoms and flare periods of symptoms that can include intensification of symptoms for hours, days, and weeks respectively.[12] Moreover, it has been suggested that there may be a common coexistence for IC/BPS with other medical conditions such as fibromyalgia, irritable bowel syndrome, chronic fatigue syndrome, chronic headaches, vulvodynia and Sjogren's syndrome suggesting a common dysregulation.[13] First-line treatment approaches are based on clinical principles as overall there is insufficient literature for an evidence-based guideline for IC/BPS. Treatments include patient education, self-care, behavioral modifications, and stress management practices. Second-line treatments include manual therapy techniques, pharmacologic therapy including urinary analgesics, non-steroidal anti-inflammatory drugs (NSAIDs), narcotic, and non-narcotic pain medications.[10] In a recent survey of complementary medicine use in patients with IC, of 1,828 subjects who completed the survey at least 84.2% had tried one form of complementary medicine that was reported to improve their symptoms. These included dietary changes (1,517, 1,329, 87.6%) (number of patients answering, number of patients reporting improvement in symptoms, percentage, respectively), application of heat or cold therapies (941, 823, 87.5), exercise (937, 611, 65.2), relaxation (763, 583, 76.4), massage therapy (493, 366, 74.2) and acupuncture (473, 260, 56.9).[14] Despite this indication of use of complementary strategies, only one study was found in the literature examining acupuncture for IC and only the abstract is available in English as the full article is written in Japanese. The study abstract reported that eight patients with refractory IC were treated with acupuncture, moxibustion, and electro acupuncture (EA) at three acupuncture points, BL32, BL33, and BL34 once a week for three months. Results showed that three of eight responders had a reduction of >2 points on their visual analog scales for bladder pain.[15] More studies are definitely needed testing acupuncture and/or EA for both male and female patients with IC/BPS.

Overactive bladder (OAB)

OAB is a symptom complex that is defined as "urinary urgency, usually accompanied by frequency and nocturia, with or without urgency urinary incontinence, in the absence of UTI or other obvious pathology".[16] Prevalence rates range from 7% to 27% in men and 9% to 43% in women. For both men and women, OAB prevalence and severity have been shown to increase with age but urge urinary incontinence is more common in women.[10] First-, second-, and third-line treatments have been suggested by the AUA. First line treatments of OAB include behavioral therapies such as bladder control strategies and fluid management with or without pharmacological agents. Second-line treatments include pharmacological agents such as oral antimuscarinic or oral B3 adrenoreceptor agonists such as solifenacin, oxybutynin, and mirabegron. Transdermal oxybutynin as a gel or patch is also available via prescription and over-the-counter. Common side effects of these medications include dry mouth and constipation. Third-line treatments include onabotulinumtoxinA injection, percutaneous electrical nerve stimulation, sacral nerve simulation, other combination therapies and acupuncture with or without percutaneous electrical nerve stimulation/EA. A number of randomized clinical trials of acupuncture have been done examining the potential role of acupuncture for the treatment of OAB symptoms. The studies have been generally well designed with regard to sample size calculations and control groups and study designs include acupuncture vs. pharmacologic therapy, acupuncture vs. sham acupuncture or acupuncture + pharmacologic therapy vs. control. There are two most recent clinical trials of interest. First is a randomized study of acupuncture vs. solifenacin. Ninety women were randomized to either acupuncture vs. solifenacin vs. placebo (sham acupuncture) for four weeks.[17] Four-day voiding diaries were required at baseline and outcomes included the International Consultation on Incontinence Questionnaire-Short Form (in Turkish) (ICIQ-SF), quality of life scores (QOL), micturition frequency, and urinary levels of nerve growth factor (NGF). NGF has been recently tested in a variety of studies to see if it may be a biomarker for symptom assessment in patients with OAB.[18] For the true acupuncture protocol the following point prescription was applied bilaterally including the points LI4, extra point *yin tang*, governing vessel 22 (DU22), CV4,

ST3, KI3, KI5, LV3, and SP6. The acupuncture protocol was applied and needling method included obtaining *de qi*. Treatment frequency was twice weekly for four weeks. The sham control was non-penetrating needles that retract into the needle handle. The solifenacin group dosing was 5 mg QD. Mean age was 38 ± 12.9. Results of the ICIQ symptom scores demonstrated a significant improvement in the acupuncture vs. sham group and the acupuncture vs. solifenacin group ($P < 0.01$, $P < 0.01$). NGF levels were reduced in both the solifenacin and acupuncture groups but not the sham group. This interesting study is limited by its short duration. Adverse events included dry mouth in the solifenacin group only. A second study examined acupuncture vs. tolterodine in 244 women. Patients were randomized to either true acupuncture vs. 2 mg tolterodine BID for four weeks.[19] Endpoints included number of episodes of urinary urgency, incontinence, daytime frequency, and voided urine volume. The acupuncture point protocol included the following four points needled bilaterally, SP6, SP9, KI3, and CV4. Results demonstrated that mean age was 57.5 ± 12.1 (18–82) 58.2 ± 11.5 (18–85) in the intervention vs. control group. At the four-week endpoint the number of urinary episodes per 24 hours decreased in both groups, as did urgency incontinence and nocturia. There were no statistically significant differences when comparing acupuncture vs. tolterodine. Adverse events included 11 reports of dry mouth in the tolterodine group vs. nine reports of needling pain the acupuncture group. This study demonstrates that both acupuncture and pharmacological treatment with tolterodine resulted in reduction of OAB in women after four weeks. This study is also limited by its short intervention period.

Two mechanistic studies are also of interest with regard to the potential mechanisms of action of acupuncture for the treatment of OAB. The first study tested sacral acupuncture needling on bladder activity related to GABAergic neurons.[20] The investigators administered sacral point acupuncture to the L5–S4 nerve roots while measuring brainstem neuronal activity and bladder pressure in anesthetized rats. Acupuncture stimulation affects the bladder when there is a period of prolonged relaxation after a bladder contraction.* Acupuncture effect was first performed in triplicate to identify responsive animals who were then used for the reminder of the study. GABAergic involvement was examined by administering a GABA antagonist and acupuncture effect was measured by comparing the mean firing rate for contraction-related cycles. Finally, cholinergic neurons were measured via immunohistochemistry after euthanization. Results revealed that acupuncture caused bladder activity as measured by the mean frequency of contraction 2.01 ± 0.89 Hz; $P < 0.05$. Acupuncture was also shown to stimulate GABAergic effects on bladder activity as demonstrated by the fact that acupuncture failed to suppress bladder contraction after administration of the antagonist bicuculline. Acupuncture also affected neurons involved in initiation, maintenance and suppression during bladder contraction as shown by immunohistochemistry vs. controls. These results suggest that acupuncture may affect both peripheral and central aspects of the nervous system. A second basic science study tested the effects of acupuncture on interstitial cells in an OAB rat model.[21] This study examined the effects of acupuncture stimulation on bladder over-activity, interstitial cells, detrusor contraction, and interstitial cell excitability. Acupuncture needling was performed near sacral nerve root points located by S2 and S4 levels respectively and points were stimulated with electricity. The results demonstrated that detrusor contraction frequency was increased in the acupuncture vs. the control group. Cystometrograms also demonstrated that there were changes in the acupuncture vs. control in bladder filling period. This study demonstrates that acupuncture stimulation suppressed bladder overactivity in an OAB rat model and affected intracellular concentration of calcium in bladder interstitial cells. This study proposes that acupuncture has both a peripherally mediated effect and a possible myogenic mechanism. In summary, there is a growing body of evidence to suggest that acupuncture and EA may have multiple physiologic mechanisms and can be a viable treatment for OAB in humans.

---

*Acupuncture Effects on Bladder Activity and State of Vigilance Through GABAergic Neuronal Systems. http://dx.doi.org/10.5772/55405

Chronic Prostatitis and Chronic Pelvic Pain

Chronic prostatitis/chronic pelvic pain syndrome (CP/CPPS) is a common urologic disease that has an incidence of affecting up to 10% of men over their lifetime.[22] Symptoms of CP/CPPS are characterized in three domains, pain (prostate, testicle, perineum, other), urinary function (frequency, urgency, dysuria) and QOL. The National Institutes of Health (NIH) collaborative has previously created a well-validated questionnaire, the NIH-chronic prostatitis symptom index (NIH-CPSI), which is a useful tool to assess symptoms and improvement to therapies at baseline and follow up time periods. A variety of treatments have been studied for men with CP/CPPS largely due to the heterogeneity in the phenotype of the condition. Currently, a multimodal treatment approach to treating CP/CPPS has been recommended and is based on the mnemonic, UPOINT. UPOINT domains include urinary symptoms, psychological dysfunction, organ-specific symptoms, infection, neurologic/systemic conditions, and tenderness of muscles.[23] Treatments for CP/CPPS include medical therapy including antibiotics, anti-inflammatories, alpha-blockers, 5α reductase inhibitors, phytotherapy, physical therapy, acupuncture, and EA. There have been numerous studies testing acupuncture in men with CP/CPPS. The most recent study analyzed 54 men with CP/CPPS and randomized them to levofloxacin 500 mg QD and ibuprofen 200mg BID for six weeks vs. true acupuncture (point prescription UB32, UB33, gall bladder 41 (GB41), LV3, LI4, SP6, SP8) twice weekly for seven weeks. The follow up was 28 weeks from baseline to assess durability and outcomes were total and subscores on the NIH-CPSI. At the follow-up period, total pain domain scores were decreased in both groups ($P<0.01$) but pain reduction was better in the acupuncture group vs. the medicine group ($P<0.05$). There were no statistically significant differences in either urinary symptoms or QOL scores between the groups although the trend showed better improvement in the acupuncture group. The mechanism of action of acupuncture for acupuncture treatment for CP/CPPS is also thought to be due to both central and peripheral nervous system effects. Based on this recent study and previous clinical trials, acupuncture has been integrated in the multimodal treatment algorithm for CP/CPPS.

Chronic Orchialgia and Epididymitis

As abovementioned, chronic orchialgia is often a subset of the CP/CPPS, however, differential diagnoses include torsion, benign masses and testicular neoplasm. However, referred pain from CP/CPPS and/or lower lumbar or sacral nerve root impingement is the most common cause of chronic testicle pain. There have been no randomized clinical trials on acupuncture for the symptom of testicle pain only.

Benign Prostatic Hyperplasia and Irritative Voiding Symptoms

Benign prostatic hyperplasia (BPH) is a histologic diagnosis and is defined as benign proliferation of epithelial and muscle cells in the prostate. The enlarged prostate frequently contributes to LUTS via bladder outlet obstruction (BOO) and/or increased smooth muscle tone and resistance.[24] Studies have shown that BPH may affect up to 50–80% of men over their lifetime.[25] Common treatments include medical and surgical approaches. Medical treatments include the use of alpha-blockers, 5α reductase inhibitors, anticholinergic agents and combination therapy. Surgical treatments include transurethral resection of the prostate, laser ablation of the prostate, transurethral needle ablation, transurethral microwave thermotherapy, and prostatectomy. In addition, LUTS may or may not be related to BPH and it is important that the clinician can distinguish prostate pathologies from those that do not have an etiology of prostatic enlargement. Studies of acupuncture for male LUTS include a study of EA vs. sham for moderate LUTS symptoms in men.[26] One hundred subjects were randomized to EA vs. sham. Inclusion criteria were men between the ages of 50 and 70 with baseline moderate LUTS as assessed by the International prostate symptom score (IPSS). The acupuncture protocol included the acupuncture points BL33 bilaterally vs. superficial non-acupuncture points. Subjects received a total of 16 treatments over four weeks. Results demonstrated that at week 7, subjects in the EA group had a statistically significant decline in IPSS scores vs. the control group ($P<0.002$). The point reduction on the IPSS was from 20.10 ± 6.52 at baseline to 12.84 ± 5.87 and study end point. Results also demonstrated that at week 18, the treatment effect remained significant. More studies are needed testing acupuncture for LUTS related to BPH.

Urinary Incontinence

Urinary incontinence (UI) includes a wide variety of LUTS and can include stress urinary incontinence (SUI), urgency urinary incontinence (UUI) and mixed urinary incontinence. There are a variety of etiologies of UI. In men, common causes of UI include radical prostatectomy, radiotherapy, aging, and BOO. In women, common causes include childbirth, aging, and previous abdominal or urogenital surgery. Common treatments include medical and surgical approaches including slings and artificial urinary sphincters. Non-medical treatments include pelvic floor physical therapy, biofeedback, and acupuncture. There are no studies examining the impact of acupuncture on male UI. In women, there are a few studies of acupuncture for UI. First, a study of EA + tolterodine vs. EA alone showed that both groups demonstrated similar and robust response rates after eight weeks.[27] 71 subjects were randomized to either EA three times a week for eight weeks or EA + 2 mg tolterodine. The acupuncture point prescription was bilateral BL32, BL35, SP6, and ST36. Results demonstrated significant reduction in UI episodes in both groups from a median decrease of four vs. three UI episodes in the EA + drug vs. EA group, respectively. Adverse events were not reported. A second pilot study assessed acupuncture or pelvic floor muscle training in women with mixed UI. This study examined feasibility of subjects being randomized to either 12 sessions of traditional Chinese medicine-style acupuncture vs. 12 sessions of pelvic floor muscle therapy vs. wait list control. Outcome measures demonstrated that recruitment was feasible and secondary outcomes showed that median scores on the International Consultation on Incontinence Questionnaire-Urinary Incontinence-Short Form (ICIQ-UI SF) were better in the acupuncture group at 5.5 (2.3–6.8) vs. physical therapy 1.0 (–3.0–4.5) vs. control 1.5 (–1.5–3.0).[28] The acupuncture treatment protocol was not accessible for review. Finally, the clinical study design for a large multicenter study has been recently published and will test the effectiveness of EA vs. solifenacin + pelvic floor muscle training for the treatment of mixed urinary incontinence. This is a large multicenter study that will randomize 500 women to receive EA three times a week for 12 weeks vs. 5 mg solifenacin + pelvic floor muscle training. The primary outcome will be the proportion of change in three-day incontinence episode frequency compared from baseline to week 12 between the two groups. The study is currently ongoing.[29]

Female Sexual Dysfunction

A study of both men and women examining the effects of acupuncture on antidepressant induced acupuncture is the only study that has been found testing acupuncture for female sexual disorders. Subjects received 12 treatments over 12 weeks and completed a number of questionnaires including the Beck Depression Inventory, the Sexual Function Visual Analog Scale (SFVAS) and the Arizona Sexual Experience Questionnaire (ASEX). The acupuncture prescription was KI3, CV4, BL23, heart 7 (HT7), and pericardium 6 (PC6). Results of the 35 subjects demonstrated that in the male participants ($n = 18$), SFVAS scores improved significantly after 12 weeks ($P = 0.001$) as did scores on the ASEX ($P = 0.017$). In females, the SFVAS trend was not significant ($P = 0.067$) and scores on the ASEX were not significant ($P = 0.384$). The authors first discuss that there is a close connection between sexual function and mental health. They also suggest that acupuncture treatment may have caused a decrease in anxiety and depression resulting in improved sexual function. Finally, they postulate that the reason for the lower response of women to acupuncture treatment may have been illness severity (baseline scores were on average higher than men) or that the women may have needed a longer treatment time. Reported side effects in the study included mild soreness due to needling, two reports of bruising, one report of muscle twitching and one report of increase emotional lability.[30] No other studies have been performed testing acupuncture for the treatment of female sexual dysfunction.

Female Pelvic Pain of Non-Gynecologic Origin

Female pelvic pain conditions of non-gynecologic origin are often encountered in urologic and urogynecologic practices and most commonly include vulvodynia. The vulvodynia (VVD) guideline defines VVD as "vulvar discomfort, most often described as burning pain, occurring in the absence of relevant visible findings or a specific, clinically identifiable, neurologic disorder".[31] A recent randomized study of 36 women tested acupuncture vs. wait list control and demonstrated a significant response in patients in the acupuncture group. The acupuncture protocol consisted of the points GV20, CV4, LI4, KI 11, ST 30, SP6, and LV3. Acupuncture frequency was two treatments twice weekly for five weeks. Outcomes included the Short-Form McGill Pain Questionnaire (SF-MPQ) and the Female Sexual Function Index (FSFI). While there was great variability between baseline subject scores (non-significant) there were significant changes between the acupuncture vs. the control group on the SF-MPG for sensory pain ($P = 0.01$), total pain ($P = 0.02$), Present Pain Intensity Scale (PPI) ($P = 0.002$) and VAS recording of pain ($P = 0.003$). For the FSFI significant improvements were shown in the sensory pain ($P = 0.003$) subscore. In addition, a small pilot study of eight women with provoked vestibulodynia (PVD) demonstrated that there were significant decreases in pain as measured by the Pain Catastrophizing Scale (PCS) after 10 acupuncture sessions over five weeks.[32]

Erectile Dysfunction

Two randomized controlled studies and a few pilot studies have demonstrated the effectiveness of acupuncture for treating erectile dysfunction (ED). The first randomized controlled study was performed in 22 subjects with psychogenic ED. Subjects were randomized to acupuncture utilizing a protocol designed to treat ED vs. acupuncture with a protocol designed to treat headache (point prescriptions were not available for review). Serum hormone levels, International Index of Erectile Function (IIEF) scores and tumescence testing were performed. Results demonstrated that there was a 68.4% improvement in the acupuncture group vs. the sham group 9% ($P = 0.0017$).[33] The second randomized study showed that acupuncture improved ED symptoms as did hypnosis but not placebo (study data not available).[34] Finally, a recent mechanistic study showed that a traditionally used acupuncture point, BL23, located at the spinous process level of L2 is in proximity with the intermediate and lateral branch of the posterior ramus of the spinal nerve at L2. This study suggests that stimulation of the acupuncture point with acupuncture needles causes stimulation of both the somatic and sympathetic nervous systems implying further mechanistic effects on its usefulness in treating urologic symptoms.[35]

Kidney Stones

There have been three studies assessing the utility of acupuncture and auricular acupressure or acupuncture on reducing pain and anxiety prior to surgical interventions for nephrolithiasis. First, Mora *et al.* utilized an auricular acupressure protocol in elderly patients prior to extracorporeal shock wave lithotripsy (ESWL). Hundred patients were randomized to auricular acupressure utilizing an auricular seed vs. sham prior to receiving ESWL at an ambulatory center. Outcome measures included a pre-intervention VAS, an anticipation questionnaire and a post-intervention VAS measuring anxiety. Auricular seeds were applied to the auricular relaxation point and remained in position until the patient was transported to the hospital. Patients in the sham group received application of an auricular seed to a non-specific point. Results demonstrated that subjects who received the true auricular seed application had significantly decreased anxiety scores vs. those in the sham group ($P = 0.001$). Subjects in the true group also had lower anticipation of pain scores (mean ± SD 57.6 ± 21.8 to 15.4 ± 9.8 and 35.7 ± 29.7 to 9.5 ± 4.1 mm VAS).[36] Two studies testing acupuncture as an anxiolytic prior to lithotripsy have also been done. Wang *et al.* performed a study of 57 patients who received pre-procedural auricular acupuncture and intraprocedural EA vs. intraprocedural sham EA. Results demonstrated that patients in the true acupuncture group were significantly less anxious as compared to those in the sham ($P = 0.020$). Patients in the true group also used less pain medicine than those in the sham group ($P = 0.040$). Alfentanil consumption was as expressed by median rate of 1 (0.6–1.6) ug/kg^{-1} minute −1 in the acupuncture group which was lower than the level in the sham group at 1.5 (0.9–2.3) ug/kg^{-1} minute −1.[37] Finally, there was a second study that assessed the utility of EA vs. sedation (tramadol + midazolam [TM]) in 35 paints undergoing ESWL. Results showed that there were no significant differences in stone size between the two groups and that VAS scores were significantly lower in the EA group vs. the TM group throughout the procedure. The acupuncture body points were BL20, BL21, BL22, BL23, and BL52, points at the levels of the thoracic vertebrae 11, 12 and lumbars 1 and 2, respectively. The electrical stimulation was given for 20 minutes and following removal of the body needles, intradermal auricular needles were embedded in *shen men*, kidney and bladder points bilaterally. Treatment with tramadol was dosed at 1.5 mg/kg and was administered 30 minutes prior to lithotripsy and the midazolam dose was 0.06 mg/kg and was administered 5 minutes prior.[38] This study was a well-designed and written study demonstrating the superiority of EA and intradermal auricular acupuncture and its ability to reduce post-procedure pain and anxiety.

Conclusion

There are a lot of urologic diseases and symptoms for which preliminary evidence exists demonstrating the effectiveness of acupuncture or EA as either a primary or part of a multidisciplinary treatment strategy. The strongest level of evidence is for the use of acupuncture as a treatment for CP/CPPS as demonstrated by the inclusion of acupuncture in the established treatment algorithm. Better-designed prospective randomized studies are needed to determine the effects of acupuncture for urologic conditions in larger numbers of patients and continued research on the mechanism side with regard to the effects of acupuncture point needling and other non-specific effects are necessary. Finally, acupuncture has minimal side effects and is a safe and tolerable non-pharmacologic procedure that can be administered to adult patients with a variety of acute and chronic medical conditions.

References

1. Foxman B. Epidemiology of urinary tract infections: incidence, morbidity, and economic costs. *Am J Med.* 2002;113 Suppl 1A:5s–13s.
2. Nicolle LE and Ronald AR. Recurrent urinary tract infection in adult women: diagnosis and treatment. *Infect Dis Clin North Am.* 1987;1(4):79–806.
3. Gupta K and Hooton T. Recurrent urinary tract infection in women. UpToDate; 2014.
4. Gupta K and Stamm WE. Pathogenesis and management of recurrent urinary tract infections in women. *World J Urol.* 1999;17(6):415–420.
5. Aydin A, Ahmed K, Zaman I, Khan MS and Dasgupta P. Recurrent urinary tract infections in women. *Int Urogynecol J.* 2015;26(6):795–804.
6. Beerepoot MA, Geerlings SE, van Haarst EP, van Charante NM and ter Riet G. Nonantibiotic prophylaxis for recurrent urinary tract infections: a systematic review and meta-analysis of randomized controlled trials. *J Urol.* 2013;190(6):1981–1989.

7. Aune A, Alraek T, LiHua H and Baerheim A. Acupuncture in the prophylaxis of recurrent lower urinary tract infection in adult women. *Scand J Prim Health Care.* 1998;16(1):37–39.
8. MacPherson H, Altman DG, Hammerschlag R, et al. Revised Standards for Reporting Interventions in Clinical Trials of Acupuncture (STRICTA): Extending the CONSORT statement. *J Evid Based Med.* 2010;3(3):140–155.
9. Alraek T, Soedal LI, Fagerheim SU, Digranes A and Baerheim A. Acupuncture treatment in the prevention of uncomplicated recurrent lower urinary tract infections in adult women. *Am J Public Health.* 2002;92(10):1609–1611.
10. Hanno PM, Burks DM, Clemens JQ, et al. Interstitial Cystitis/Bladder Pain Syndrome: American Urological Association. 2014. Available on: https://www.auanet.org/education/guidelines/ic-bladder-pain-syndrome.cfm.
11. Hanno P and Dmochowski R. Status of international consensus on interstitial cystitis/bladder pain syndrome/painful bladder syndrome: 2008 snapshot. *Neurourol Urodyn.* 2009;28(4):274–286.
12. Warren JW, Brown J, Tracy JK, Langenberg P, Wesselmann U and Greenberg P. Evidence-based criteria for pain of interstitial cystitis/painful bladder syndrome in women. *Urology.* 2008;71(3):444–448.
13. Aaron LA and Buchwald D. A review of the evidence for overlap among unexplained clinical conditions. *Ann Intern Med.* 2001;134(9 Pt 2):868–881.
14. O'Hare PG, 3rd, Hoffmann AR, Allen P, Gordon B, Salin L and Whitmore K. Interstitial cystitis patients' use and rating of complementary and alternative medicine therapies. *Int Urogynecol J.* 2013;24(6):977–982.
15. Katayama Y, Nakahara K, Shitamura T, et al. Effectiveness of acupuncture and moxibustion therapy for the treatment of refractory interstitial cystitis. *Hinyokika Kiyo.* 2013;59(5):265–269.
16. Haylen BT, de Ridder D, Freeman RM, et al. An International Urogynecological Association (IUGA)/International Continence Society (ICS) joint report on the terminology for female pelvic floor dysfunction. *Neurourol Urodyn.* 2010;29(1):4–20.
17. Aydogmus Y, Sunay M, Arslan H, Aydin A, Adiloglu AK and Sahin H. Acupuncture versus solifenacin for treatment of overactive bladder and its correlation with urine nerve growth factor levels: a randomized, placebo-controlled clinical trial. *Urol Int.* 2014;93(4):437–443.

18. Kim JC, Park EY, Seo SI, Park YH and Hwang TK. Nerve growth factor and prostaglandins in the urine of female patients with overactive bladder. *J Urol.* 2006;175(5):1773–1776; discussion 1776.

19. Yuan Z, He C, Yan S, Huang D, Wang H and Tang W. Acupuncture for overactive bladder in female adult: a randomized controlled trial. *World J Urol.* 2015;33(9):1303–1308.

20. Wang H, Tanaka Y, Kawauchi A, Miki T, Kayama Y and Koyama Y. Acupuncture of the sacral vertebrae suppresses bladder activity and bladder activity-related neurons in the brainstem micturition center. *Neurosci Res.* 2012;72(1):430–449.

21. Feng QF, Hou YH, Hou WG, Lin ZX, Tang KM and Chen YL. The effects of acupuncture on bladder interstitial cells of cajal excitability in rats with overactive bladder. *Evid Based Complement Alternat Med.* 2013;2013:261217.

22. Nickel JC, Downey J, Hunter D and Clark J. Prevalence of prostatitis-like symptoms in a population based study using the National Institutes of Health chronic prostatitis symptom index. *J Urol.* 2001;165(3):842–845.

23. Nickel JC and Shoskes DA. Phenotypic approach to the management of the chronic prostatitis/chronic pelvic pain syndrome. *BJU Int.* 2010;106(9):1252–1263.

24. McVary, KT RC and Avins AL. American Urological Association Guideline: Management of Benign Prostatic Hyperplasia (BPH). Advancing Urology; 2010.

25. McVary KT. BPH: epidemiology and comorbidities. *Am J Manag Care.* 2006;12(5 Suppl):S122–S128.

26. Wang Y, Liu B, Yu J, Wu J, Wang J, Liu Z. Electroacupuncture for moderate and severe benign prostatic hyperplasia: a randomized controlled trial. *PLoS One.* 2013;8(4):e59449.

27. Jin C, Zhou X, Pang R. Effect of electroacupuncture combined with tolterodine on treating female mixed urinary incontinence. *J Wound Ostomy Continence Nurs.* 2014;41(3):268–272.

28. Solberg M, Alraek T, Mdala I, Klovning A. A pilot study on the use of acupuncture or pelvic floor muscle training for mixed urinary incontinence. *Acupunct Med.* 2016;34(1):7–13.

29. Liu B, Wang Y, Xu H, et al. Effect of electroacupuncture versus pelvic floor muscle training plus solifenacin for moderate and severe mixed urinary incontinence in women: a study protocol. *BMC Complement Altern Med.* 2014;14:301.

30. Khamba B, Aucoin M, Lytle M, *et al.* Efficacy of acupuncture treatment of sexual dysfunction secondary to antidepressants. *J Altern Complement Med.* 2013;19(11):862–869.
31. Haefner HK, Collins ME, Davis GD, *et al.* The vulvodynia guideline. *J Low Genit Tract Dis.* 2005;9(1):40–51.
32. Curran S, Brotto LA, Fisher H, Knudson G, Cohen T. The ACTIV study: acupuncture treatment in provoked vestibulodynia. *J Sex Med.* 2010;7(2 Pt 2):981–995.
33. Engelhardt PF, Daha LK, Zils T, Simak R, Konig K, Pfluger H. Acupuncture in the treatment of psychogenic erectile dysfunction: first results of a prospective randomized placebo-controlled study. *Int J Impot Res.* 2003;15(5):343–346.
34. Aydin S, Ercan M, Caskurlu T, *et al.* Acupuncture and hypnotic suggestions in the treatment of non-organic male sexual dysfunction. *Scand J Urol Nephrol.* 1997;31(3):271–274.
35. Umemoto K, Saito T, Naito M, *et al.* Anatomical relationship between BL23 and the posterior ramus of the L2 spinal nerve. *Acupunct Med.* 2016;34(2):95–100.
36. Mora B, Iannuzzi M, Lang T, *et al.* Auricular acupressure as a treatment for anxiety before extracorporeal shock wave lithotripsy in the elderly. *J Urol.* 2007;178(1):160–164; discussion 164.
37. Wang SM, Punjala M, Weiss D, Anderson K and Kain ZN. Acupuncture as an adjunct for sedation during lithotripsy. *J Altern Complement Med.* 2007;13(2):241–246.
38. Resim S, Gumusalan Y, Ekerbicer HC, Sahin MA and Sahinkanat T. Effectiveness of electro-acupuncture compared to sedo-analgesics in relieving pain during shockwave lithotripsy. *Urol Res.* 2005; 33(4):285–290.

Chapter 7

Physical Therapy Evaluation and Manual Therapy Treatment Strategies for Pelvic and Urologic Disorders

Jannafer Vande Vegte, MSPT, PRPC, BCB-PMD

*Physical Therapist, Pelvic Floor Specialist,
Pelvic Floor Biofeedback Certified, Spectrum Health,
Grand Rapids MI 49512*

Bridgid Ellingson, PT, DPT, OCS

*Owner, Lakeview Physical Therapy, P.C.
4001 N. Ravenswood Ave., Suite
402 Chicago, IL 60613*

Amy Stein, DPT, BCB-PMD

*Owner/Founder
Beyond Basics Physical Therapy, LLC
110 E 42nd St Suite #1504 NY, NY 10017*

Manual therapy is noted as the physical treatment of the body to treat a variety of musculoskeletal disabilities. This practice involved the manipulation of the joints in combination with kneading of the tissues. The use of this therapy can have positive results in patients experiencing pelvic and urological disorders. This chapter will address the different disorders and how the tackle them utilizing these techniques.

Introduction

Manual therapy for the pelvic floor is both an art and a science. As an art, the provider needs to be skilled enough to discern valuable information from manual assessment and use fingers and hands that both assess and treat dysfunctional tissue, at times simultaneously. As a science, the provider must have a concrete grasp of the evidence-based research presented in the literature, terminology, assessment and treatment techniques to apply as well as knowledge about the various diagnoses that are associated with pelvic floor dysfunction. The provider must also possess an understanding of pain science and theories. Beyond providing skilled manual therapy techniques to manage pelvic pain, another key component is to provide education about high-level pain physiology[1] as well as education about healthy bowel, bladder, and sexual function.[2]

Thiele was one of the first researchers to describe the benefit of manual therapy for overactive pelvic floor dysfunctions. In his paper in 1963, he described using massage techniques to the posterior pelvic floor to cure coccygodynia in 91% of his study population.[3] However, it was not until 1994 that internal vaginal and rectal assessment and treatment were added to the Guide to Physical Therapy Practice.[4] The field of pelvic health has been growing rapidly since that time and both the art and the science of manual therapy for the pelvic floor continue to evolve.

The myofascial system of the pelvic floor comprises three distinct muscle layers and specific fascial tissues. The muscles are (see Figure 1) composed of predominately slow twitch muscle fibers with a smaller percentage of fast twitch muscle fibers. The slow twitch muscle fibers provide the endurance for pelvic support and continence throughout the day while the fast twitch fibers provide power for support and assistance in urethral sphincter closure when there is a large increase in intra-abdominal pressure like a cough or sneeze.

There are several functions of the pelvic floor muscles defined in the literature. The pelvic floor muscles are responsible for providing support for the pelvic organs, namely, the bladder, uterus, and rectum in women, and the bladder and rectum in men. The muscles play a role in controlling the opening and closing of the pelvic passageways for elimination and intercourse.[5,6] Sexual arousal and orgasm rely in part on healthy, functioning pelvic floor muscles.[5,7] The pelvic floor along with the transverse abdominus, diaphragm and multifidi muscles assists in trunk stability and load transfer.[8–10] When there is a strong urge or bladder contraction, pelvic floor activation can help quiet detrusor activity.[11]

There are muscles that work synergistically with the pelvic floor. The striated urethral sphincter contracts synergistically with the gluteals, the adductors and the pelvic floor, but not with the abdominal muscles.[12] The pelvic floor and abdominals

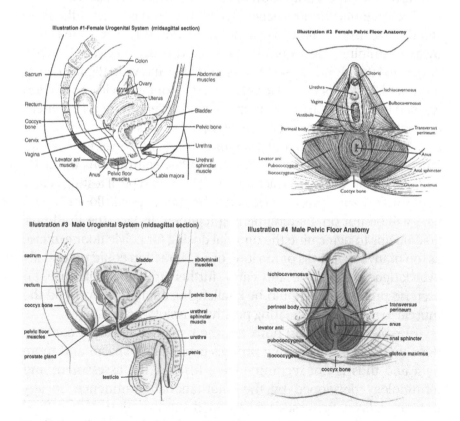

Figure 1:   Illustrations of male and female urogenital systems and pelvic floor anatomy; images with permission from heal pelvic pain by Amy Stein DPT.

contract synergistically, more specifically the transverse abdominus and the inferior fibers of the internal obliques.[10] Healthy functioning of the pelvic floor is thus dependent upon an entire system of neuromuscular control and not just one muscle group.

The pelvic floor muscles attach to the bones of the pelvis. Research has shown that compared to controls, women with pelvic pain were much more likely to have both asymmetries in the alignment of the pelvic bony landmarks and significantly more tender points throughout the pelvic floor muscles and abdominal muscles.[13] Women with visceral disorders such as painful bladder syndrome (PBS) and endometriosis are also more likely to have tenderness in the pelvic floor muscles.[13,14] Alternately, it has also been shown that women who are not experiencing pelvic pain do not have pain upon palpation of their pelvic floor muscles.[15]

The quantification of pelvic floor function has been difficult to standardize. In the clinic, pelvic floor function is typically measured by an examining finger inserted into the vagina or rectum. Laycock developed the PERFECT scheme as a reliable and valid digital assessment tool. P stands for power generated by one muscle contraction (graded from 0 to 5). E is how many seconds of endurance the patient can hold at the same muscle power, up to 10. R is how many repetitions of the same number of seconds at the same power level before fatigue (up to 10) and F tests number of fast contractions up to 10. ECT stands for "every contraction timed."[16] This type of testing is very appropriate in patients with weak or underactive pelvic floor muscles who will be put on a strengthening regimen. In fact, the PERFECT grade helps to determine the optimal dosing for pelvic floor exercise as too many repetitions or too long of a contraction could potentially over fatigue the muscle and cause further problems. Likewise, an exercise prescription should be challenging enough to overload the muscle to the point of creating positive physiological changes.

In patients with pain however, the repetitive maximal contractions involved in this testing process could cause spasm and more pain and thus is not recommended. Instead, the assessment and terminology developed by the International Continence Society can be utilized for assessment and documentation. Pelvic floor contraction is described as strong, normal, weak or non-functional meaning no palpable change of muscle activity. The muscle's ability to relax is then graded as full, partial or non-relaxing. Patients who present with pelvic floor muscle pain and overactivity often present as weak and partial or non-relaxing. There are often trigger points present upon palpation. It should be noted again that a healthy, normal functioning pelvic floor should not be painful to touch.[15] FitzGerald and Kotarinos went on to further describe a condition they termed the "short pelvic floor." In this case, the pelvic muscle is non-relaxing because of structural changes in the muscle which have caused adaptive tissue shortening.[17] This muscle condition needs to be addressed through stretching and lengthening to enact a change on the collagen and elastin that make up the muscle and fascia that surrounds it. Other authors have shown positive effects using biofeedback to build awareness and learn muscle function. Via a computer screen a patient can see whether their muscle is active or relaxed and learn improved control and coordination of their pelvic floor.[18]

Pelvic floor under activity may result in pelvic dysfunction. Often the provider observes thin atrophied muscle with low tone. There may be a wider vaginal vault, and laxity around the perineal body and anus. There is not usually pain with palpation but pain can be present if there are areas of adhesions, muscle overactivity or scar tissue combined with laxity. Pelvic floor muscle activation may be weak and or poorly coordinated and endurance is usually low. Patients may be struggling with incontinence of urine, stool or gas and pelvic organ prolapse. Pelvic floor under activity may be associated with increased parity, pudendal nerve denervation, and connective tissue laxity.[19] Incontinence can affect men, women, and even children. Stress urinary incontinence (SUI) is a condition where urine leaks as a result of increased abdominal pressure such as a cough, laugh, lift or sneeze. Stress incontinence can be associated with dysfunctional pelvic floor and abdominal wall muscles, breathing disorders, pelvic organ prolapse, prostatectomy, etc.[8,9,20] Today, many people have now heard of strengthening their pelvic floor (Kegel exercises) when they have urine leakage, and popular magazines and internet may give advice on certain exercises. Unfortunately, only 50% of women in one study performed the contraction correctly when given written instructions and 25% of those women experienced worsening symptoms with repeated incorrect Kegels, which highlights the potential need for more direct intervention.[21]

While automatic reactions of the pelvic floor muscles occur in most people when position changes or intra-abdominal force increases, automatic reactions can be delayed or absent in some people.[10] Research has shown that there is a correlation between lower back pain and breathing disorders with SUI and decreased automatic muscle functioning.[9] Janis Miller taught patients with stress incontinence to pre contract their pelvic floor muscles prior to a cough or sneeze or other situation that caused leakage and called this strategy "The Knack." She found many women were able to prevent leakage by improving the timing of their pelvic floor contraction.[22]

In a study by Swift, pelvic organ prolapse is a common condition seen in 66% of 1,000 women aged 18–84. Cystocele or decreased support around the bladder or anterior vaginal wall is seen most commonly. The development of prolapse is associated with multiparity, smoking, advanced maternal age, length of second stage of labor, instrumented vaginal birth, weight of baby, activities that increase intra-abdominal pressure such as constipation and repetitive or heavy lifting, and advancing age.[23] While prolapse is a dysfunction or failure of the connective tissue support of the pelvic organs, it is often seen along with pelvic floor dysfunction. The pelvic floor muscles play an important role in protecting the pelvic fascia from excessive stretch and tissue strain.[6] To that end one would expect to see underactive pelvic floor muscles in patients with prolapse, but at times this is not the case and the pelvic floor muscles are overactive or shortened in response to trying to compensate for the poor support of the connective tissue. Hagen treated women with stages 1 and 2 prolapse with pelvic floor muscle training and lifestyle advice and 63% reported improved function while 45% actually improved their prolapse stage.[24]

Urge Incontinence, Urgency, and Frequency Syndrome

Urge incontinence, urgency and frequency are often seen in tandem with dysfunctional pelvic floor muscles. Urgency occurs when bladder contracts strongly, often with a trigger such as cold exposure or putting one's key in the door lock, and this may result in accidental loss of urine. Trigger points in the pelvic floor and abdominal wall can create feelings of urgency and frequency for patients.[25,26] At times, pelvic floor muscle strengthening is appropriate to aid in closure of the urethra as well as reflexively inhibit the detrusor;[11] however, this can further shorten the pelvic floor muscles. The provider must rely on the physical exam and not just the patient's subjective complaints to provide the correct treatment for this condition. It is also important to note that stress, consumption of acidic, caffeinated, and alcoholic food and drink, low estrogen levels in women, constipation, drug side-effects and other factors can play a role in urgency, frequency and urge incontinence as well.

Pelvic floor over-activity may be a component of chronic pelvic pain (CPP). Often women who are experiencing CPP have higher rates of additional pelvic pain diagnoses such as interstitial cystitis/painful bladder syndrome (IC/PBS), endometriosis, vulvodynia/provoked vestibulodynia.[27] CPP is also experienced co-morbidly with conditions such as migraines, chronic fatigue, fibromyalgia, and TMJ disorder.[28] Peters highly recommends addressing pelvic floor muscle dysfunction first when it is found co-morbidly with IC/PBS and especially if palpation of the pelvic floor produces bladder symptoms.[14] It is important to note that other triggers may be associated with pelvic pain such as trauma, pelvic surgery, severe life stressors, and PTSD.[14]

Women with CPP were also shown to have a larger percentage of abuse history, PTSD, and HPA axis dysfunction (hypothalamus, pituitary, adrenal gland).[29] While men with chronic pelvic pain/chronic prostatitis also have higher rates of anxiety and depression, Ku warns that it is impossible to determine if chronic pain creates physiological disturbance or if stress and mental distress affect somatic structures.[30]

Overactive bladder/hypertonicity: Treatment is required for any pain or dysfunction in the abdomen, back, thigh, hip, genital, or pelvic region and/or any pain associated with urination or defecation, or with sexual activity related to the musculoskeletal system.

Fenton points to recent data collected by functional MRI to theorize why we see certain patterns in chronic pain patients. The limbic system has shown to be involved in a subset of women with multiple pelvic pain diagnoses, who had a history of abuse, did not respond in a typical fashion to standard treatment, showed minimal pathology in involved organs and whose pain was recurrent in nature. MRI data revealed over-activity in the anterior cingulate cortex, hippocampus and amygdala, areas of the brain responsible for emotion and memory formation among other functions. These parts of the brain were sending abnormal efferent signals to both the pelvic muscles and the pelvic viscera which created tonic contraction in these structures. The tonic contraction then fed back information into the limbic system and a cycle is created. Foster postulates that treating both the limbic system dysfunction as well as the muscular and visceral dysfunction could lead to better outcomes. He warns though that without "full disruption of the central hyper vigilance pelvic floor dysfunction and pelvic pain will reoccur". Treating the muscle dysfunction is one way to break the cycle of limbic system over-activity, as the afferent signals from the pelvic floor to the brain would decrease. Other suggested treatments that shut down the afferent arm of this cycle were Botox, trigger point injections, medications such as amytryptaline and acupuncture. Surgery and further trauma to involved tissues is not recommended but patients treated with pelvic floor therapy alone are likely to relapse.[27] It is important in clinical decision making to determine if there could be limbic system dysfunction in patients with CPP.

Vanderveen found other emotional associations with the pelvic floor. Women with and without vaginismus (an unconscious reflexive contraction of the pubococcygeus muscle often impairing vaginal penetration) were shown four movie clips while the tension in the pelvic floor was monitored. Scenes that depicted threat or fear were associated with increased pubococcygeus muscle activity in all women, not just those with vaginismus. Vanderveen concluded that the vaginistic response is a normal body response to fear and threat. Brauer assessed healthy volunteers as well as women with surface dyspareunia (pain at the opening of the vagina) and monitored them for symptoms of sexual arousal while watching erotic film clips. The women were told they had a 60% chance of getting a painful stimulus while watching the films. Interestingly, pain-related fear inhibited arousal in all women.[31] These studies show the importance of neurologic functioning, current perceptions and past experiences in treating women with CPP.

Sexual Function and Dysfunction in Men and Women

The pelvic floor muscles are proposed to play a role in sexual function, in arousal and orgasm.[32] Both underactivity and overactivity of the muscles in women and men may lead to sexual dysfunction. Pelvic pain, trigger points or pelvic floor muscle overactivity can result in pain with sexual activity and or orgasm. During arousal in women, the anterior vaginal wall lengthens and the uterus moves superiorly.[33] These changes may be important for the woman's body to prepare for penetration. However, when there is the fear of pain, arousal is impaired and these changes might not take place.[31] Men with overactive pelvic floor dysfunction may experience concurrent sexual dysfunction including ejaculatory pain, decreased libido, erectile dysfunction, premature ejaculation, and ejaculatory difficulties.[26]

Commonly underactive muscles are seen with poor arousal and orgasm in women.[7] and poor erectile and ejaculatory function in men. Likewise, if a woman is afraid of leaking it will be difficult to relax and enjoy sexual intimacy. Prolapse can cause discomfort and is linked to decreased levels of sexual health and poor genital body image.[22] But surgical corrections for bladder or pelvic organ dysfunction can also have unpleasant side effects in terms of blood flow, anatomy and sensation and create problems with arousal, orgasm, and dyspareunia.[32]

Pelvic floor muscle intervention has been helpful in the treatment of erectile and ejaculatory dysfunctions in men.[34] When pelvic floor therapy was administered to women suffering from prolapse and lower urinary tract dysfunction, sexual functioning scores also improved.[12] In men and women with sexual dysfunction and concurrent pelvic floor disorders manual treatment has been helpful in reducing pain and restoring sexual function.[26,34] In addition, Anderson *et al.* researched that treatment of a group of men with pelvic pain with trigger point release and relaxation significantly improved sexual outcome scores.[26]

Evaluation of Pelvic Floor Musculoskeletal Dysfunction

The evaluation and treatment of pelvic floor disorders can be complex. Multiple areas and functions of the body need to be assessed and treated in a skilled and thoughtful way. The patient's symptoms must be continually reassessed while providing and progressing treatment. This chapter contains a summary of evaluation strategies and manual therapies commonly used by providers but does not represent an exhaustive list.

Observation

Observing your patient begins immediately. How is he or she sitting during the interview process? Do you note any gait deviations? While discussing his or her history, what can you observe about their posture or even their personality? Posture in sitting and standing is important to note. It is common for individuals with pelvic pain to have postural deviations such as increased lumbar lordosis and increased anterior pelvic tilt.[35] Diane Lee has coined the terms upper chest gripper for those who are dominant in upper external oblique activity, back gripper for those who are overactive in thoracic paraspinals and butt gripper describing those who do not relax their gluteal muscles. She goes on to inform us that these motor control issues may affect the body in a myriad of ways. Chest grippers may not be utilizing their diaphragm correctly leading to dysfunctional changes in intra-abdominal pressure which may affect the pelvic organs and pelvic floor negatively. Back grippers may have postural pain especially with standing. The increased activity of the spinal extensors may put undue pressure through the joints of the spine while also limiting the activity of the anterior abdominals. Butt grippers will not move correctly at the hip joint putting more pressure on the anterior hips. They also may have postural pain as they will tend to sit in a posterior tilt position flexing the normal lumbar curve.[8]

A standing assessment should also include a functional movement assessment. Squatting can reveal much about a person's musculoskeletal deficits and compensations such as the inability to achieve optimum gluteal and pelvic floor length as well as ankle, knee, hip, lumbar and even thoracic restrictions that influence pelvic mechanics. Squatting has been shown to be an integral component of a comprehensive pelvic treatment program.[36] Standing on one leg for 30 seconds is a functional test for gluteus medius endurance.[37] If the contra lateral hip drops in single leg stance or if the standing leg internally rotates and adducts further muscle testing may reveal weakness or poor neuromuscular coordination. If the function of the hip stabilizers is impaired this may result in either concurrent weakness or over activity of the pelvic floor as it attempts to compensate for poor hip stability.

Range of Motion: Musculoskeletal System

Range of Motion (ROM) assessments are especially important at the hips, pelvis, sacrococcygeal joint and spine because these areas impact the pelvic region directly. ROM of the spine can be performed standing while the hips and pelvis can be evaluated functionally in standing and then formally if needed in supine or prone. Recently there have been studies showing that hip labral tears can decrease hip ROM and can cause irritation to the hip rotators, the pelvic floor muscles and nerves, and create chronic vulvar pain.[38,39]

Strength: Core and Lower Extremity Muscles

Measuring strength can also be done functionally and with specific muscle testing. It is important to assess the strength and motor recruitment patterns of the trunk and the lower extremities. The Active Straight Leg Raise (ASLR) is a clinical test to unveil poor compensation patterns in translating load from the LE to the trunk. The patient is asked to lie supine and raise one leg about six inches, then the other. The patient notes any difficulty or differences sided to side. The therapist is watching for asymmetries, pelvic or spinal instabilities. Then the therapist can use his or her hands to stabilize the patient while the leg is lifted again. If the movement is easier or improved, the therapist can infer what muscles might not be working properly.[8]

Palpation: muscle

Attention should be given to the muscles of the trunk and abdomen, hips and thighs, and the three layers of pelvic floor musculature. The practitioner is assessing for pain, muscle tone, trigger points and tender points as well as areas of myofascial or visceral restriction. Mense made an interesting study in the difference between trigger points and tender points and concluded "Signs and symptoms of MTrPs: (1) palpable nodule, often located close to the muscle belly, (2) often single, (3) allodynia and hyperalgesia at the MTrP, (4) referral of the MTrP pain, (5) normal pain sensitivity outside the MTrPs, (6) local twitch response, (7) local contracture in biopsy material, (8) peripheral mechanism probable. Signs and symptoms of MTrPs: (1) no palpable nodule, (2) location often close to the muscle attachments, (3) multiple by definition, (4) allodynia and hyperalgesia also outside the MTrPs, (5) enhanced pain under psychic stress, (6) unspecific histological changes in biopsy material, (7) central nervous mechanism probable. The multitude of differences speak against a common etiology and pathophysiology."[40] A muscle with a trigger point or points will be in a shortened position and will lack the appropriate length tension ratio of its sarcomeres to function well.[41] The presence of multiple trigger points may be an indicator of centralized sensitization of pain.

Palpation: Joints

The spine, pelvic, and hip joints are assessed for areas of hyper or hypo mobility that may be of clinical relevance. Foot and ankle mobility may also be assessed as Ingrid Nygaard found that college athletes with hypomobile feet were more likely to also have SUI.[42]

Although position tests of the sacroiliac joint have been shown to have poor inter-rater reliability movement, tests combined with provocation tests have been shown to have higher confidence in determining sacroiliac involvement.[43] As mentioned earlier, research has shown that women with pelvic floor dysfunction are more likely to have pelvic girdle asymmetries.[13]

Palpation: Nerves

Consideration also should be given to the nerves of the pelvic region in both men and women. A patient's history may direct the provider to look more closely for specific neuralgia or possible, but not very common, nerve entrapment. The nervous system is a complex and dynamic system in its own right. Peripheral nerves can be influenced by tension in fascia and muscles and by changes in blood flow. Scar tissue, inflammation and adhesions can restrict mobility and function of peripheral nerves.[44]

The pudendal nerve is the main nerve to the pelvis arising from sacral nerve roots S2-4. It is composed of sensory fibers (80%) and motor fibers (20%) and is the only peripheral nerve to have connections to both the autonomic and somatic nervous systems. Involvement of this nerve may then be influenced by changes in the autonomic nervous system and patients may experience symptoms such as increased heart rate, sweating, decreased colon motility and decreases blood pressure and blood flow when the nerve is stimulated. It is the only innervation to pelvic floor muscle layers 2 and 3 and shares innervation with the levator ani nerve at layer 3. It takes a tortuous route through the pelvis, which has proven to vary in many patients;

diving between the sacrotuberous and sacrospinous ligaments, winding around the ischial spine, traveling along the medial aspect of the ischial tuberosity at Alcock's canal before reaching the perineum, where it branches into three sections: the dorsal nerve to the clitoris or penis, perineal and inferior rectal branch. Palpating along the nerve pathway especially at the common sites of restriction and reproducing symptoms is an important clinical finding. Pudendal neuralgia can be commonly seen along with pelvic floor muscle dysfunction. The pudendal nerve is vulnerable to compression and injury from sitting, trauma to the pelvis, pelvic inflammation and adhesions, as a result of surgery including vaginal mesh surgeries, bike riding, and other causes. Symptoms may be unilateral or bilateral and present at various points along the distribution of the nerve. Symptoms may include pain with sitting or biking, pain reproduced by wearing tight underwear or restrictive clothing, bladder and bowel symptoms such as urgency, frequency, urinary retention or hesitancy and constipation. There may be burning and shooting or sharp pain, itching, tingling, or cold sensations in the groin, buttocks, abdomen, or legs. A pelvic nerve block may be helpful both diagnostically and as a mode of pain relief.

Other nerves are vulnerable to injury from back, abdominal and hip injuries and dysfunctions. The genitofemoral, ilioinguinal and iliohypogastric nerves arise from the thoracolumbar junction and wind around the psoas muscle (the genitofemoral actually runs through the muscle) into the lower abdominal and pelvic regions. These nerves are vulnerable to irritation caused by thoracolumbar dysfunction, psoas tension and trigger points, entrapment by mesh of inguinal or abdominal hernia repairs and certain bladder slings, abdominal surgeries and scars, connective tissue and abdominal wall trigger points. The obturator nerve arises from the lumbar nerve roots 2 through 4 and innervates the adductor and the obturator externus muscle. It may be injured during vaginal mesh surgeries, vaginal birth, and pelvic trauma. Injury to this nerve causes difficulty with gait caused by weakness of adduction and internal rotation. The lateral femoral cutaneous nerve arises from L2 and L3 and travels posterior to the psoas, anterior to the quadratus lumborum and iliacus and under the inguinal ligament. It can be entrapped or injured by hyper hip flexion, pregnancy and compression along the nerve.[45]

Pelvic and Genital Exam

The pelvic portion of the exam is typically performed with the patient in the lithotomy position with legs supported. It is important that the patient is as relaxed and comfortable as possible to get an accurate assessment. The provider should thoroughly explain the purpose and steps of the examination before touching the patient and be sure to document verbal or written consent. Even then the provider should continue a dialogue with the patient during the exam letting the patient know when and where to expect touch or pressure.

The exam begins with observation. The provider observes the vulva in women and the perineum in men looking for skin changes, hair loss, lesions, and muscle tension. A sensory exam may be performed next. A moistened cotton swab may be used to provide light touch along the perineum in men, and the vestibule and vulva to test for allodynia and hyperesthesia that is often found in women with provoked vestibulodynia or vulvodynia. Pain intensity and location are recorded. The literature describes using a clock template to describe the position of testing like numbers of a clock around the vestibule, and pain scales range from 0 to10 or 0 to 3. Documentation may read "pain of 2/3 at 4 and 8 o'clock."[27] A cotton swab may also be used for reflex testing at the clitoris and anus and sensory changes along the dermatomes.

Muscle function is assessed visually at first. The patient is asked to contract, relax, and push out or bulge the pelvic floor while the provider is analyzing motor control, accessory muscle use, breathe holding as well as total excursion of the pelvic muscles.

Next, a palpation exam uses a gloved finger to first assess the superficial or layer 1 muscles of the pelvic floor, which include the bublospongiosis, ischiocavernosis, and superficial transverse perineal. These muscles are not assessed for strength with the Laycock scale but can be assessed for pain, tone, and contractibility.

If the patient is appropriate for and consents to an internal examination, a gloved and lubricated finger is placed into the vagina or rectum. If it is appropriate, strength and endurance can be assessed using the Laycock model, otherwise contraction, relaxation and bulging can be graded using ICS terminology. Palpation should include layer two muscles (compressor urethra, urethrovaginal sphincter and deep transverse perineal) for pain, tone, and contractibility. Layer three muscles include the pubococcygeus, iliococcygeus, coccygeus, and obturator internus, as well as important fascial tissues, the ATLA (arcuate tendon levator ani) and ATFP (arcuate tendon fascia pelvis). The provider's examining finger should trace each muscle from origin to insertion looking for pain, tender or trigger points, tone and contractibility. At times, detailed palpation reveals a tear or avulsion of one of the pelvic floor muscles which is associated with higher rates of prolapse and poorer surgical outcomes.[46]

A prolapse exam is also important for women. In physical therapy practice, the anterior and posterior vaginal walls are assessed. The therapist inserts a gloved finger into the vagina so that the hymenal remnants are at the level of the therapist's finger knuckle. To test the anterior wall, the finger pushes gently posterior while the finger splints anteriorly to test the posterior wall. The patient is asked to give maximal pressure bulging the tissue inferiorly. The therapist notes where on the finger the tissue protrudes to and grades this protrusion appropriately (Grade 1:1 cm or more above the hymenal ring, Grade 2: between one cm above or below the hymenal ring, Grade 3: more than 1 cm below the hymenal ring and Grade 4: complete extrusion).[23] Physicians performing prolapse measurements may use a Sims speculum. Physical therapy has been shown to be helpful to reduce both the grade and the symptoms of genital organ prolapse in women.[24]

It may be important to assess the anal sphincters and puborectalis muscle rectally in women and men. Childbirth tears and episiotomies may have created scar tissue or nerve damage to the fibers of the external anal sphincter limiting the muscles ability to contract circumferentially to provide continence of gas and stool. The puborectalis and anal sphincters may be found to be non-relaxing and have pain, tone and trigger points in cases of elimination disorders.

There are also times when an internal exam either vaginally or rectally is either contraindicated (as with active infection), not consented to, or otherwise inadvisable. In this case, the provider may be able to still gain valuable information about pelvic floor function by visual inspection and external palpation. Layer one muscles are easily palpated with an external approach. The pubococcygeus and iliococcygeus muscle bellies may be palpated and assessed through the gluteus maximus fibers between the anus and the ischial tuberosity. The pubococcygeus is more medial and closer to the anus and the iliococcygeus more lateral. The provider, making sure to observe for substitution of the gluteal muscles, can ask for a pelvic floor contraction to ascertain correct hand positioning and depth of palpation. The obturator internus can be palpated externally in supine, hook lying, or side lying (testing the superior or inferior leg depending on the providers preference). The muscle is found on the medial aspect of the ischial tuberosity. With a flat hand the provider applies pressure fingers first to the space between the anus and the ischial tuberosity. When the hand has sunk into the ischiorectal fat, palpation is directed laterally into the obturator internus. Asking the patient to gently, isometrically externally rotate the hip will provide feedback to the provider. These muscles can be assessed for motor performance, pain, tension and trigger points and appropriate treatment can be applied.

The history and physical assessment give important evidence for determining the correct treatment choice for each patient. The provider must recognize and appreciate the various layers of dysfunction that may be present and plan appropriately to address each in turn. For example, pelvic floor overactivity may be driven by a hip labral tear, which can then refer pain to the vulvar area.[38,39] In cases of endometriosis, vulvodynia or IC, a patient may develop trigger points and pelvic floor dysfunction as a result of clenching in an unconscious attempt to protect the abdomino-pelvic region.[47] Also, chronic lower back pain may lead to muscle imbalances that affect the length tension relationship in the muscles of the lower back, hips and pelvic area. Some patients will benefit from multiple providers addressing various aspects of their disorder. Working in conjunction with a team has been shown to be advantageous especially for complex diagnoses.[48]

Treatment

Strain counter strain

Strain and Counter strain is a gentle soft tissue manipulation technique developed by Dr. Lawrence Jones D.O. and Randy Kusenose, PT, OCS, over a 40-year period. This technique can be effective in treating pain, muscle spasm, tightness and decreased ROM. It is painless and has no side effects and can be applied to many different muscles. Dr. Jones describes his technique as a "passive positional procedure that places the body in a position of greatest comfort, thereby relieving pain by reduction and arrest of inappropriate proprioceptor activity that maintains somatic dysfunction". The position of maximal comfort is referred to as the mobile point and is typically the maximally shortened position of the muscle. The provider palpates for a tender point in the involved muscle which is then monitored during the positioning of the body until the tender point is no longer painful. This position is held for 90 seconds. It is imperative that the position is released slowly and with care especially during the first 15° of movement. This technique can be very effective when applied to the peripheral muscles, and the patient can be taught the therapeutic positioning for home.[49]

Strain counter strain can be applied to internal and external pelvic floor muscles singularly and concurrently to the abdominal, pelvic, hip, lumbar, and sacral tissues. The approach may address general muscle layers and specific muscles. It can be utilized to treat painful entry into the vaginal or anorectal canals for patients with vaginismus, dyspareunia, anismus. The practitioner can address each muscle involved, empower the patient with self or partner included home strategies that are pain-free and effective.[8,50]

Myofascial Trigger Point Release

Myofascial trigger point release is defined as the release of tender points or hyperirritable spots, usually within taut bands of skeletal muscle or in the muscle fascia which is painful on compression and can give rise to characteristic referred pain, motor dysfunction, and autonomic phenomena.[51] When palpated a trigger point (as opposed to a tender point) refers pain, often in a predictable and reproducible pattern. Trigger points can develop from direct trauma to the tissue or by repeated microtraumas. When palpating the tissue the provider is aware of a taut band in the muscle, discerning this by strumming across the muscle fibers, using the thumb and index finger to compress the tissue, or with pressure applied directly into deeper muscles of the body. A muscle that has a trigger point is typically shortened, weak, demonstrates poor coordination and decreased ROM, and has increased tone. As a result, the muscle or the surrounding muscles have to work harder to perform their usual functions and muscle dysfunction may propagate.[47]

The following is a list of muscles that are commonly seen to have trigger points or muscle dysfunction in patients with pelvic pain conditions: pelvic floor muscles, obturator internus, coccygeus, abdominals, gluteals, adductors, piriformis, quadratus lumborum, paraspinals, iliotibial band/tensor fascia lata, quadriceps, and hamstrings.[51] Pelvic floor muscle trigger points may refer pain to the bladder, rectum, genitals, lower back, hip, perineum, coccyx, and abdomen. They may also reproduce feelings of urgency in the bladder or rectum.[25,26]

When a trigger point is located, a provider may use a variety of techniques to eliminate the pain arising from this tissue and restore its length, coordination, and function. If the pain is too intense to treat directly, strain counter strain may be a good option. Direct approaches may include ischemic pressure and contract/relax/stretch. Ischemic pressure involves applying pressure directly to the trigger point. This should be done to patient tolerance as the patient needs to be able to relax the muscle being treated. The theory is that direct, localized pressure will prevent blood flow to the trigger point. When the pressure is released, fresh blood will flood the tissue carrying away irritating tissue exudates and bringing nutrients for the dysfunctional tissue. Stretching the muscle after using ischemic pressure is important to restore tissue length.[51]

Contract/relax stretching can also be used to release trigger points and treat overactive or shortened muscles with or without trigger points. This technique utilizes the neurological reflex that occurs after a muscle is contracted, there is a brief period when greater relaxation is induced after the contraction. To apply this principle in the pelvic floor, the provider may utilize a gloved finger in the vaginal or anal canal and rest the length of the finger against the vaginal or anal side wall. The provider asks for a small, submaximal contraction of the pelvic floor. The patient holds this contraction for approximately 5 seconds. As the patient relaxes the muscles, the provider uses gentle pressure to take up the slack in the tissue and hold it for a gentle stretch. The contract/relax/stretch process can be repeated several times as long as the tissue is responding in a positive way. Patients can be taught to perform this technique at home with a finger or a dilator.

Soft Tissue Mobilization

At times, a patient may present with a muscle that is not just overactive, but actually shortened and possibly fibrosed.[17] These muscles may present with painful tender points or trigger points, have poor excursion and function, and need to be lengthened as part of the therapeutic process. A variety of tissue mobilization strategies such as strumming or stripping along or across the muscle fibers, kneading the muscle, and providing oscillations or vibration to the tissues can be employed by the provider to manipulate, release and stretch the dysfunctional muscle and connective tissue. The provider or the patient can apply stretching strategies to the muscle to continue tissue remodeling to promote length of the shortened structures.

Connective Tissue Mobilization

Connective Tissue Mobilization is a direct tissue technique that mobilizes connective tissue restrictions between layers of tissue. This techniques is thought to improve connective tissue integrity, increase blood flow, and reduce pressure on the nerves in the region.[52] Subcutaneous panniculosis is reduced as the provider glides his or her thumbs along the restricted tissue while the fingers feed a roll of skin toward the thumbs (see Figure 2). The sensation the patient feels when the tissue is restricted, may be pinching or scratching or nail digging. The sensation increases in intensity in more restricted areas. The patient may complain of pain or bruising during and after the session. If pain is a barrier, the technique should still be performed but may be performed more slowly and gently to help with patient tolerance. The provider should address restrictions from superficial to deep, and from caudal to cephalad. Adverse reactions could include fainting and palpitations if there is a strong sympathetic response. Patient tolerance should be monitored[50] and the provider should monitor and document changes to skin texture, color (often there is a strong histamine response) temperature and elasticity. The results of this technique are also thought to be cumulative with each session building upon the last.[52,53]

Neural Mobilization

The nervous system is a continuous system composed of neurons as well as connective tissue that surrounds the nerves to protect it and help it glide through surrounding tissues. The nervous

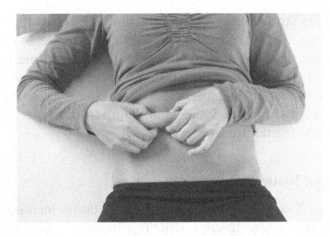

Figure 2: Illustration of connective tissue mobilization technique.

system should slide, glide, bend, stretch, and move as we move do. Anything that interrupts the normal movement of neural tissues — a sacroiliac dysfunction, a bulging disk, a muscle spasm, or swollen compartments — will cause pain, will decrease blood supply in the nerve and may displace the myelin sheath. Trauma, inflammation, constriction, chronic muscle tension, surgery can restrict the physiological motion of the nerves and create pain. It is important for the provider to know the anatomy of the major nerves to the pelvis and consider potential restriction if a patient's subjective and objective findings lead to this consideration. It should be noted that before treating the nerves directly the muscles and connective tissue in the area must be adequately treated. Often, this treatment alone will be beneficial to the patient and relieve symptoms. Prendergast describes mobilizing the branches of the pudendal nerve with manual techniques of stabilizing the perineal tissues near the groin and then stretching and skin rolling along the three main branches of the pudendal nerve. If symptoms are not fully resolved, nerve glides are performed in a very gentle, mobilizing but not necessarily stretching motion. An example of a pudendal nerve glide could be gently bulging the pelvic floor and could be progressed to a repeated, slow, wide leg squat. If this is tolerated well by the patient the technique can be progressed to include a gentle stretch like adding cervical flexion to a wide leg squat.[52,53]

Myofascial Release

The myofascial system comprises a thin layer of connective tissue fibers that are mostly collagen that give structure, stability and separation to the muscles and internal organs of the body. Fascia can be classified according to region and function into superficial fascia located under the skin, deep fascia which is around muscles, bones, nerves and blood vessels and visceral fascia which supports the organs. When the system is functioning well, fascia helps to reduce tension in the tissues, provide support as well as ease of glide and motion for the organs and vessels.[54] When fascia is disrupted by inflammation, injury, scarring or adhesions, it will not function properly and chronic pain can ensue.[55]

With myofascial release the provider uses his or her hands to locate areas of poor mobility in the fascia and applies a gentle force either in the direction of the restriction for a direct approach, or applies force opposite the restriction in the direction of slack for an indirect approach. The indirect approach is often utilized when a patient has great pain or when pain is acute, for example, after a recent surgical procedure.[55]

Visceral Mobilization

Although this will be discussed in depth in another chapter, it is important to mention the importance of this therapy in assessing and treating pelvic dysfunction. Visceral Mobilization consists of skillfully applied, gentle, manual therapy techniques directed at identifying and correcting imbalances in the mobility and motility of the organs. These imbalances may have been created by trauma, inflammation, surgery, scar tissue, adhesions, etc. and can negatively affect the healthy functioning of organs and the systems to which they belong.[44]

Coordination/Strength Training/Manual Feedback

Often a provider's hands, patient positioning and verbal instruction can be utilized to help a patient identify or improve motor functioning and control. Because a patient cannot see their pelvic floor contracting like they could their quadriceps or bicep, it is often difficult for them to find the correct recruitment pattern to appropriately contract and relax this muscle group. Some patients because of their injury, their pain or simply their life experience tend to have less body awareness than others. Providing manual feedback in the form of simple palpation can help a patient identify a muscle. Adding resistance can help recruit a stronger contraction of a muscle. Tapping, stroking or a quick stretch to the muscle are other strategies providers can use to help up train muscle performance. Stretching the muscle, adding resistance, vibration, traction, inhibitory tendon pressure, fast brushing, light touch, and slow stroking are all examples of techniques that are available to facilitate or inhibit muscle to help normalize muscle tone.[50]

Biofeedback, which will be discussed in detail in a subsequent chapter, is also a helpful tool to the patient and the practitioner.

Joint Position and Mobility

Because of the interrelationship between joint and muscle function and networked nerve supply in and around the pelvis and common innervation points between structures, joint hypo and hyper mobility as well as asymmetries in joint positions are often found in men and women with pelvic dysfunctions.[13,35] The provider should evaluate and treat any abnormalities in the spinal column including joints and disks, the hip joint capsule and ligaments, and the joints and ligaments of the pelvic girdle.[8,35]

There are many different strategies to correct joint position and improve articular coordination and movement. Muscle energy is one strategy employed by providers. In muscle energy techniques, the body is positioned in such a way that the joint to be treated is aligned into the restriction. The patient is asked to then contract the shortened muscles gently usually for 5 seconds. This contraction creates a reflex relaxation in the tight muscles so slack can be taken up and the joint repositioned until the next barrier is felt. This process is repeated several times until the barriers or movement restrictions are improved. It may be important to then provide some movement reeducation to ensure that the muscles around the joint are coordinating through the improved ROM of the joint or joints.[56]

Direct mobilization is another option for improving joint position and mobility. Varied pressure, oscillations, or vibrations are applied to a restricted joint to create a mechanical effect and can be applied to any of the joints of the body but mainly to the spine, pelvis, and hips in patients with pelvic disorders. Normalizing joint function in terms of ROM, stability, proprioception is as imperative as correcting soft tissue dysfunction.[8]

One should note that advanced joint manipulation may also play a role in pelvic treatment, however, these techniques require specialized training.[8]

Manual Lymph Drainage

Pelvic congestion syndrome (PCS) is another dysfunction that may be either a primary cause of pelvic pain or exist along with other diagnoses or dysfunctions. Pelvic congestion occurs when venous or lymphatic fluids accumulate in the pelvic regions. Symptoms include CPP that is worse with prolonged standing, prolonged sitting, pain during and after (for up to 24 hours), urinary frequency, painful periods and venous varicosities.[57] Imaging of pelvic veins is helpful to diagnose this problem. Regarding treatment of PCS Umranikar notes, "Although many medical and surgical approaches to this clinical entity are in part effective, the management continues to be challenging and often requires a more holistic and multidisciplinary approach."

The lymphatic system has the job of returning the fluid from other tissues of the body to the blood stream. All the lymphatic vessels from the lower pelvis and chest, lower limbs, and abdomen, empty into the thoracic duct. The fluid that travels through this duct is called lymph, which consists mostly of white blood cells and is similar to blood plasma.

Lymphedema is a chronic condition that can occur anywhere in the body where the body's ability to transport fluid along lymph pathways is impaired.[50] It can be primary or secondary and is usually seen after cancer operations, radiation, with tumors and infections.

Providers may use manual therapy to assist in lymph and vascular drainage within the pelvis. Manual lymph drainage massage is performed by using light strokes to promote the flow to lymph fluid toward open channels and away from blockages. Practitioners who are skilled in this treatment should have at least 135 hours of training in a certification program.[50]

Myofascial Decompression or "Cup Therapy"

Myofascial Decompression, also known as Cup Therapy, is based on ancient medical techniques with roots in cultures from around the world including Hippocratic physicians in ancient Greece.[58] Physical therapists most often employ plastic cups with a manual hand pump to create a negative pressure over an area presenting with myofascial restrictions (see Figure 3). The goal is to increase blood flow and nutrient exchange; release tonic, tight, facilitated muscles; and traction out deep connective tissue. It also relieves pain by acting as a counterirritant. The neurophysiologic response results in an increase in endogenous opioids or endorphins that affect the limbic system and brain stem, and enkephalins that affect the central nervous system.[59] For patients presenting with pelvic pain, myofascial decompression can be used to mechanically alter restricted connective tissue; release trigger points, and to mobilize C-section and other scars. Careful placement of cups over the ischial tuberosities the adductors and adjacent to the coccyx can be an effective to way to mobilize fascia that is continuous into the pelvic floor. It may be possible to use this technique to mechanically decompress a nerve that is being compromised by surrounding or adjacent tissue.[60] Myofascial decompression should be used in conjunction with neuromuscular re-education to result in improved movement patterns and posture.

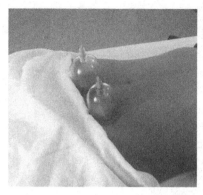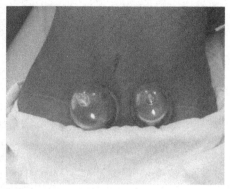

Figure 3: Illustration of myofascial decompression or "Cup Therapy"; Photo with permission from Bridgid Ellingson.

Dry Needling

Dry needling (DN) therapy is a skilled intervention that uses a thin filiform needle to penetrate the skin and stimulate underlying myofascial trigger points, muscular, and connective tissue restrictions for the management of neuromusculoskeletal pain and movement impairments.[4] DN to treat myofascial trigger points (TrPs) involves multiple advances of a needle into the muscle at the region of a trigger point to elicit a localized twitch response which is modulated by the central nervous system (see Figure 4).[61] DN also normalizes the chemical milieu and pH of skeletal muscle[11,62] and restores the local circulation. The first part of Moseley's three part approach to managing the individual specific pain neuromatrix advises that "nociceptive mechanisms that contribute to threatening information should be treated".[63] DN of TrPs reduces local and referred pain and can be used as a part of a comprehensive treatment approach to managing abdomino-pelvic pain.

Patients with abdomino-pelvic pain may benefit from DN of involved muscles of the pelvic girdle and abdomen including the muscles of the hip and thigh as well as the ishiocavernosus, bulbospongiosus/bulbocavernosus, superficial and deep transverse perineal, pubococcygeus, iliococcygeus, and the coccygeus muscles.[64] In addition, the segmental spinal root should also be

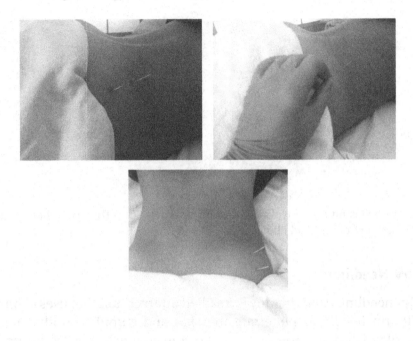

Figure 4: Illustration of DN technique; photos with permission from Bridgid Ellingson.

assessed and treated if appropriate. DN should be performed in conjunction with neuromuscular re-education and patient education to improve movement patterns and posture.

Abdominal/Intestinal Massage

Abdominal/intestinal massage is a strategy used to promote healthy functioning of the intestinal tract. Bowel dysfunction is often seen concurrently with pelvic disorders such as pelvic pain and bladder problems. After reviewing literature from 1999 to the present, Sinclair writes, "Studies have demonstrated that abdominal massage can stimulate peristalsis, decrease colonic transit time, increase the frequency of bowel movements in constipated patients, and decrease the feelings of discomfort and pain that accompany it. There is also good evidence that massage can stimulate peristalsis in patients with post-surgical ileus."[65] Visceral massage was shown to be effective in decreasing post-surgical ileus in rats.

Emly describes this protocol for abdominal massage for constipation. The procedure begins with a gentle stroking from inferior to superior up the abdominal wall. If the patient has reflux or a hiatal hernia the initial stroking direction should be reversed. Gentle stroking continues then along the dermatome of the vagus nerve, over the iliac crests, and along the pelvis toward the groin. Effleurage is next, following the normal transit of stool along the large intestine: starting at the ascending colon and moving superiorly, laterally across the transverse colon and inferiorly along the descending colon. Kneading inferiorly along the descending colon and superiorly along the ascending colon with a firmer, palmar or finger approach (if it is appropriate for the patient) is the next step. Kneading helps to break up and propel fecal matter. Effleurage is again performed as previously stated. The next technique is a gentle, relaxing transverse stroke over the entire abdomen. Lastly, vibration is performed along the abdomen to release any flatulence. Many providers use a simplified version of this protocol both in the clinic and to teach patients self-treatment. The ILU massage uses circular massage strokes and begins with massaging inferiorly along the descending colon (I), then along the transverse colon and back down the descending colon (L), lastly moving superiorly along the ascending colon all the way through to the descending colon (see Figure 5).[20]

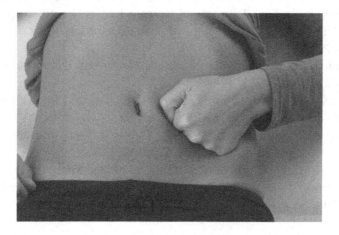

Figure 5:   Illustration of abdominal massage.

Pelvic floor muscle function can range in scope from normal, non-functioning, weak, non-relaxing/overactive, short or contractured. Pelvic floor muscle dysfunction can exist on its own or concurrently with visceral, articular, neural or myofasical disorders. Addressing pelvic floor dysfunction whether primary or secondary should be a first line of treatment for patients struggling with pelvic pain, sexual dysfunction, and elimination disorders. Because the pelvic floor functions as part of a complete system, a systemic evaluation of the trunk, pelvis and hip joints, muscles, nerves and connective tissue should be performed and treatment applied as indicated. Manual therapy techniques have an important role in improving function and decreasing pain. They are considered safe and effective when applied by a skilled provider as part of a comprehensive treatment program. Many techniques can also be adapted and self-administered by the patient as part of a self-care program.

References

1. Hilton S and Vandyken C. The Puzzle of Pelvic Pain — A Rehabilitation Framework for Balancing Tissue Dysfunction and Central Sensitization, I: Pain Physiology and Evaluation for the Physical Therapist. *J Womens Health Care*. 2011;35(3):103–113.
2. Berzuk K. The Pelvic Floor Muscle: the Link Between Bladder, Bowel, and...Sex? A Review of Current Pelvic Therapy Approaches for Diagnosis and Treatment of Sexual Disorders. *Curr Sex Health Rep*. 2014;6(3):192–200.
3. Thiele GH. Coccygodynia: cause and treatment. *Dis. Colon Rectum*. 1963;6:422–436.
4. American Physical Therapy Association. *Guide to Physical Therapist Practice. Phys Ther*. 2001;81(1):9–746.
5. Kegel AH. Sexual functions of the pubococcygeus muscle. *West. J. Surg. Obstet. Gynecol*. 1952;60(10):521–524.
6. Ashton-Miller JA, Howard D and DeLancey JOL. The Functional Anatomy of the Female Pelvic Floor and Stress Continence Control System. *Scand. J. Urol. Nephrol. Suppl*. 2001;35:1–7.

7. Lowenstein L, Gruenwald I, Gartman I and Vardi Y. Can stronger pelvic muscle floor improve sexual function? *Int Urogynecol J.* 2010;21(5):553–556.
8. Lee D. *The Pelvic Girdle: An Integration of Clinical Expertise and Research.* 4th ed: Churchill Livingstone Elsevier; 2011.
9. Smith M, Coppieters M and Hodges P. Postural activity of the pelvic floor muscles is delayed during rapid arm movements in women with stress urinary incontinence. *Int Urogynecol J.* 2007;18(8):901–911.
10. Hodges PW, Sapsford R and Pengel LHM. Postural and respiratory functions of the pelvic floor muscles. *Neurourol. Urodyn.* 2007;26(3): 362–371.
11. Shafik A and Shafik IA. Overactive bladder inhibition in response to pelvic floor muscle exercises. *World J. Urol.* 2003;20(6):374–377.
12. Bo K, Berghmans B, Morkved S and Van Kampen M. *Evidence-Based Physical Therapy for the Pelvic Floor.* Philadelphia, PA: Churchill Livingstone Elsevier; 2007.
13. Tu FF, Holt J, Gonzales J and Fitzgerald CM. Physical therapy evaluation of patients with chronic pelvic pain: a controlled study. *Am. J. Obstet. Gynecol.* 2008;198(3):272.e271–272.e277.
14. FitzGerald MP, Anderson RU, Potts J, *et al.* Randomized Multicenter Feasibility Trial of Myofascial Physical Therapy for the Treatment of Urological Chronic Pelvic Pain Syndromes. *J Urol.* 2009;182(2): 570–580.
15. Kavvadias T, Pelikan S, Roth P, Baessler K and Schuessler B. Pelvic floor muscle tenderness in asymptomatic, nulliparous women: topographical distribution and reliability of a visual analogue scale. *Int Urogynecol J.* 2013;24(2):281–286.
16. Laycock J and Jerwood D. Pelvic Floor Muscle Assessment: The PERFECT Scheme. *Physiotherapy.* 2001;87(12):631–642.
17. FitzGerald MP and Kotarinos R. Rehabilitation of the short pelvic floor. I: Background and patient evaluation. *Int Urogynecol J.* 2003;14(4):261–268.
18. Koh CE, Young CJ, Young JM and Solomon MJ. Systematic review of randomized controlled trials of the effectiveness of biofeedback for pelvic floor dysfunction. *Br. J. Surg.* 2008;95(9):1079–1087.
19. Fletcher E. Differential diagnosis of high-tone and low-tone pelvic floor muscle dysfunction. *J Wound Ostomy Continence Nurs.* 2005; 32(3S):S10–S11.

20. Bishoff JT, Motley G, Optenberg SA, *et al.* Incidence of fecal and urinary incontinence following radical perineal and retropubic prostatectomy in a national population. *J Urol.* 1998;160(2):454–458.

21. Bump RC, Hurt WG, Fantl JA and Wyman JF. Assessment of Kegel pelvic muscle exercise performance after brief verbal instruction. *Am. J. Obstet. Gynecol.* 1991;165(2):322–327; discussion 327–329.

22. Zielinski R, Miller J, Low LK, Sampselle C and DeLancey JOL. The relationship between pelvic organ prolapse, genital body image, and sexual health. *Neurourol. Urodyn.* 2012;31(7):1145–1148.

23. Swift S, Morris S, McKinnie V, *et al.* Validation of a simplified technique for using the POPQ pelvic organ prolapse classification system. *Int Urogynecol J.* 2006;17(6):615–620.

24. Hagen S, Stark D, Maher C and Adams E. Conservative management of pelvic organ prolapse in women. *Cochrane Database Syst Rev.* 2006(4):Cd003882.

25. Wise D and Anderson R. *A Headache in the Pelvis: A new understanding and treatment for the prostatitis and chronic pelvic pain syndromes.* Occidental, CA: National Center for Pelvic Pain; 2003.

26. Anderson RU, Wise D, Sawyer T and Chan CA. Sexual dysfunction in men with chronic prostatitis/chronic pelvic pain syndrome: improvement after trigger point release and paradoxical relaxation training. *J Urol.* 2006;176(4):1534–1539.

27. Haefner HK, Collins ME, Davis GD, *et al.* The vulvodynia guideline. *J. Low. Genit. Tract Dis.* 2005;9(1):40–51.

28. Aaron LA, Burke MM and Buchwald D. Overlapping conditions among patients with chronic fatigue syndrome, fibromyalgia, and temporomandibular disorder. *Arch. Intern. Med.* 2000;160(2):221–227.

29. Heim C. Abuse-related posttraumatic stress disorder and alterations of the hypothalamic-pituitary-adrenal axis in women with chronic pelvic pain. *Psychosom. Med.* 1998;60(3):309–318.

30. Ku JH, Kim SW and Paick J-S. Quality of life and psychological factors in chronic prostatitis/chronic pelvic pain syndrome. *Urology.* 2005;66(4):693–701.

31. Brauer M, ter Kuile MM, Janssen SA and Laan E. The effect of pain-related fear on sexual arousal in women with superficial dyspareunia. *Eur. J. Pain.* 2007;11(7):788–798.

32. Pauls RN and Berman JR. Impact of pelvic floor disorders and prolapse on female sexual function and response. *Urol. Clin. North Am.* 2002;29(3):677–683.

33. Schultz WW, van Andel P, Sabelis I and Mooyaart E. Magnetic resonance imaging of male and female genitals during coitus and female sexual arousal. *BMJ*. 1999;319(7225):1596–1600.
34. Rosenbaum TY. Pelvic floor involvement in male and female sexual dysfunction and the role of pelvic floor rehabilitation in treatment: A literature review. *J Sex Med*. 2007;4(1):4–13.
35. Baker PK. Musculoskeletal origins of chronic pelvic pain. Diagnosis and treatment. *Obstet Gynecol Clin North Am*. 1993;20(4):719–742.
36. Petros PP and Skilling PM. Pelvic floor rehabilitation in the female according to the integral theory of female urinary incontinence: First report. *Eur J Obstet Gynecol Reprod Biol*. 2001;94(2):264–269.
37. Bewyer DC and Bewyer KJ. Rationale for Treatment of Hip Abductor Pain Syndrome. *Iowa Orthop J*. 2003;23:57–60.
38. Coady D, Futterman S, Harris D, Shah M and Coleman SH. The relationship between labrum tears of the hip and generalized unprovoked vestibulodynia. Paper presented at: International Society for the Study of Vulvovaginal Disease World Congress. Edinburgh, Scotland; 2009.
39. Prather H, Spitznagle TM and Dugan SA. Recognizing and treating pelvic pain and pelvic floor dysfunction. *Phys. Med. Rehabil. Clin. N. Am*. 2007;18(3):477–496, ix.
40. Mense S. Differences between myofascial trigger points and tender points. *Der Schmerz*. 2011;25(1):93–104.
41. Gordon AM, Huxley AF and Julian FJ. The variation in isometric tension with sarcomere length in vertebrate muscle fibres. *J Physiol*. 1966;184(1):170–192.
42. Nygaard IE, Glowacki C and Saltzman CL. Relationship between foot flexibility and urinary incontinence in nulliparous varsity athletes. *Obstet. Gynecol*. 1996;87(6):1049–1051.
43. Cibulka MT and Koldehoff R. Clinical usefulness of a cluster of sacroiliac joint tests in patients with and without low back pain. *J. Orthop. Sports Phys. Ther*. 1999;29(2):83–89; discussion 90–82.
44. Barral JP and Mercier P. *Visceral Manipulation*. Seattle, WA: Eastland Press; 2005.
45. Hollis MH, Lemay DE and Jensen MP. Nerve entrapment syndromes of the lower extremity. *Medscape Reference*. 2010.
46. Model AN, Shek KL and Dietz HP. Levator defects are associated with prolapse after pelvic floor surgery. *Eur J Obstet Gynecol Reprod Biol*. 2010;153(2):220–223.

47. Reissing ED, Brown C, Lord MJ, Binik YM and Khalife S. Pelvic floor muscle functioning in women with vulvar vestibulitis syndrome. *J. Psychosom. Obstet. Gynaecol.* 2005;26(2):107–113.

48. Davis K and Kumar D. Pelvic floor dysfunction: a conceptual framework for collaborative patient-centred care. *J. Adv. Nurs.* 2003;43(6): 555–568.

49. Jones L and Kusunose R. Originators of the Strain Counterstrain Technique. Available on: http://www.jiscs.com/Article.aspx?a=11 (Accessed July 10, 2014).

50. Carrière B, Markel Feldt C. *The Pelvic Floor.* Thieme; 2006.

51. Travell J and Simons D. *Myofascial Pain and Dysfunction,* Vol. 1: *The Trigger Point Manual, The Upper Extremities.* Baltimore, MD: Williams and Wilkins; 1983.

52. Butler DS. *The Sensitive Nervous System.* Adelaide, Australia: Noigroup Publications; 2000.

53. Prendergast S and Rummer E. De-Mystifying Pudendal Neuralgia: A Physical Therapist's Approach. 2009; Chicago, IL.

54. Benjamin M. The fascia of the limbs and back — a review. *J. Anat.* 2009;214(1):1–18.

55. Barnes JF. Myofascial release approach. *Massage* 2006.

56. Greenman PE. *Principles of Manual Medicine.* Baltimore: Williams & Wilkins; 1989.

57. Umranikar A, Cheong Y. Pelvic Congestion Syndrome. *Chronic Pelvic Pain.* Blackwell Publishing Ltd.; 2011;65–70.

58. Christopoulou-Aletra H and Papavramidou N. Cupping: An Alternative Surgical Procedure Used by Hippocratic Physicians. *The Journal of Alternative and Complementary Medicine.* 2008;14(8): 899–902.

59. Da Prato C and Kennedy C. Myofascial Decompression Techniques: A Movement Based Myofascial Course; 2009.

60. FitzGerald MP and Kotarinos R. Rehabilitation of the short pelvic floor. II: Treatment of the patient with the short pelvic floor. *Int. Urogynecol. J. Pelvic Floor Dysfunct.* 2003;14(4):269–275; discussion 275.

61. Hong CZ. Lidocaine injection versus dry needling to myofascial trigger point. The importance of the local twitch response. *Am. J. Phys. Med. Rehabil.* 1994;73(4):256–263.

62. Shah JP and Gilliams EA. Uncovering the biochemical milieu of myofascial trigger points using in vivo microdialysis: An application

of muscle pain concepts to myofascial pain syndrome. *J. Bodyw. Mov. Ther.* 2008;12(4):371–384.

63. Moseley GL. A pain neuromatrix approach to patients with chronic pain. *Man. Ther.* 2003;8(3):130–140.
64. Sandalcidi D and Dommerholt J. Deep dry needling of the hop, pelvis and thigh muscles. In: Dommerholt J, Fernandez-de-las-Penas C, eds. *Trigger Point Dry Needling.* Elsevier; 2013:133–150.
65. Sinclair M. The use of abdominal massage to treat chronic constipation. *J. Bodyw. Mov. Ther.* 2011;15(4):436–445.

Chapter 8

Adjunct Modalities for Physical Therapy

Lila Bartkowski-Abbate, PT, DPT, MS, OCS, WCS, PRPC Owner/Director

New Dimensions Physical Therapy, Manhasset, NY 11030

Allison Ariail, PT, DPT, CLT-LANA, BCB-PMD, PRPC Owner/Director

Inspire Physical Therapy and Wellness Lone Tree, CO 80124; Parker, CO 80138

Andrea Wood, PT, DPT

Staff Physical Therapist New Dimensions Physical Therapy Manhasset, NY 11030

An alternative method to treating a variety of urological disorders is the use of a physical modality. These modalities can range from the use of heat to sound waves all in an effort to produce a desired effect for the patient such as reducing pain or increasing the flow of blood into a region of the body. This chapter will discuss the use of these modalities along with the concept of biofeedback, which is the process of bringing awareness to the patient and to the provider. Research in this area has proven biofeedback can bring about successful results in a variety of urological disorders.

Introduction

A part of a treatment plan to treat a urological ailment may include the use of a physical modality. A modality is the use of a physical agent such as heat, cold, electricity, sound waves, or laser to produce a desired effect. The effects could include decrease in inflammation, increase in blood flow, decrease in pain, or change in elasticity of the tissues.

Additionally, the use of surface electromyography (sEMG), biofeedback, and ultrasound imaging may provide further assessment information to allow the clinician to quantify results, and rule out pathology. They can also be used to enhance treatment by providing the patient with more information and insight into their body as they perform an activity.

Modalities

Heat and ice

Cryotherapy or cold packs are used to decrease pain by several mechanisms. When ice is applied to tissues, vasoconstriction occurs. This slows circulation to the tissues, which decreases the amount of swelling in the area, therefore decreasing pain.[1] Cold treatment also slows nerve conduction rates, decreasing the number of pain messages to the brain. For pelvic pain patients, cold treatment can alleviate the constant burning and other pain sensations. This can be applied by placing a small ice pack to the perineal area, or freezing a water or witch hazel filled pad and then placing it on the perineum. Other methods of applying cold include filling a condom with water and freezing it, or placing a tool, such as a dilator or TheraWand, in the freezer. These cold instruments can then be used for vaginal or perineal application. These should not be placed directly against the skin or placed directly into the vagina.

Heat also can decrease pain via several mechanisms. Heat causes vasodilation to occur. Vasodilation causes increased blood flow to the area which increases the flow of oxygen and nutrients to the area, helping to speed the rate of healing. The elasticity of muscles and tissues is improved after the application of heat, this can aid in the healing of scars. Additionally, heat stimulates sensory receptors located in the skin. This will result in less transmission of pain signals, and can relieve some of the pain. Heat for pelvic pain can be applied in several ways including a dry heating pad, a moist heating pad, immersion in a warm bath, therapeutic ultrasound, and short wave diathermy. Compared to heating pads, studies have shown that the temperature of muscles increases more via the immersion method.[2]

Ultrasound and electrical stimulation variants

Therapeutic ultrasound uses sound waves to heat the area. A transducer with gel is used to transmit the ultrasound waves into the body. The maximum effect will be 2–5 cm depth depending on the frequency used. Ultrasound can be used to aid in muscle and scar tissue elasticity, and is often used to treat perineal scars following childbirth or surgery.[3]

Transcutaneous electrical stimulation, or TENS, uses low voltage electrical current to reduce pain and improve symptoms of urinary and fecal incontinence. Electrodes are placed on the skin that then produce a current through the body. The current travels on the skin and along the nerves to block pain signals from reaching the brain. TENS has been shown to be effective in decreasing pain for individuals suffering chronic prostatitis and chronic pelvic pain (CPP).[4]

Interferential therapy uses a higher frequency electrical current compared to TENS, which allows it to reach greater depths. Four electrodes are placed on the skin in such a way that two currents are crossing each other over the area with pain. When these two currents intersect each other, interference occurs, which blocks pain signals at the spinal cord level. Interferential therapy has been used to treat painful bladder syndrome and CPP.

Neuromuscular electrical stimulation (NMES) is also used to strengthen weakened pelvic floor muscles using a vaginal or rectal sensor. The exact mechanism of how it strengthens the muscles is currently unclear. The stimulation may produce a contraction of the pelvic floor muscles. Using the stimulation frequently can then improve the strength. Protocols vary but traditionally 15–20 minute sessions are recommended one to two times a day. NMES has been used for many years by clinicians, however, the evidence for this is not strong and more research is needed to prove the effectiveness.[5]

High voltage pulsed galvanic stimulation (HVPGS) is another form of electrical stimulation that has shown benefits in patients pelvic pain. Unlike other forms of electrical stimulation that uses alternating currents, HVPGS uses direct current with higher voltages and very short pulse duration. This allows deeper penetration without damaging the tissues and allowing for more comfort. A rectal probe is placed in the anus to deliver the current. HVPGS has been shown to successfully treat levator ani syndrome and rectal pain.[6]

Additional modalities

Short wave diathermy is the use of high frequency electromagnetic waves to generate heat inside the body. It has been shown as an effective treatment for patients with pelvic inflammatory disease.[7]

Cold laser therapy or low level laser therapy uses low intensity infrared light that does not produce heat. Laser therapy enhances healing by decreasing inflammation, increasing circulation, and improving nerve function.

Biofeedback

Biofeedback is a modality that gives consciousness to the patient and knowledge to the provider. This offers an educational and positive outcome to the patient which brings empowering information to the patient. In general, biofeedback can be any type of modality that brings awareness to anything that the patient can control. It can be in simple forms of respiration and heart rate. The main use in physical therapy is skeletal muscle awareness and control. Biofeedback can give the patient information on where to target their strength, to understand how the wrong muscle can be working too much and how a specific muscle cannot be firing at all.

During physical therapy sessions, feedback can come in various forms. In the women's health arena, it can range from low back pressure cuffs for transversus and multifidus firing, vaginal cones, external sensors along the perineum, and rectal balloons for internal anal sphincter training along with internal vaginal and rectal sensors. These modalities help treat patients, women, men, and children, with complaints of various pelvic floor disorders such as urinary incontinence, fecal incontinence, chronic constipation, and pelvic pain. The awareness of muscle tone and function helps the provider to instruct the patient to either work on up-training (making the muscles stronger), down-training (learning to relax the muscles) or coordination training (teaches the patient to use their muscles in an appropriate sequence). There are many advantages of using biofeedback. Biofeedback can help increase motivation and allows the patient to be less passive in their treatment. It also has non-invasive options and recordings can be taken in various positions other than supine which carryover to functional tasks such as preventing urinary incontinence when carrying a laundry basket or when lifting packages. Biofeedback recordings through machines or use of external supplies can increase awareness of muscular changes that a patient may not be able to feel and muscle patterns may be observed that are not available with plain sight.

Biofeedback for the pelvic floor principles

Biofeedback using internal vaginal and rectal sensors or surface electrodes measures muscle action potentials through the electrodes or sensors to help to increase muscular coordination with the addition of auditory and visual feedback. The electrodes and sensors record the change in microvolts over the muscle fiber membrane as it starts contraction and relaxes. The therapist can also assess resting tone, quick contractions, and endurance of the pelvic floor muscles more in depth. It is important to note biofeedback using electrodes and sensors does not directly indicate muscle strength, force, tension, or muscle length or spasm, but rather it records a chain of events that cause muscle actions to occur.[8] It can also be used in conjunction with transvaginal electrical stimulation, an additional modality that uses non-painful electrical stimulation through electrodes placed in the vagina to help the pelvic floor muscles contract and relax.

Electrodes can be placed intravaginally, in the anus, (internal vaginal or rectal sensors) or around the anus on the surface (external biofeedback pads). Intravaginal and intrarectal sensors are much more specific and give accurate reading to the internal pelvic floor muscles, whereas external pads give overflow to gluteus maximus activity. The benefits of using sEMG are that they can be used in pregnant/post-partum patients, post-surgery, and in pelvic pain patients that may not tolerate internal sensors. They are also inexpensive and come in disposable form. Surface electrodes tend to be about 1 cm or smaller. They can be placed on the perianal region with gloved hands at 3 and 9 o'clock while the patient is sidelying, 1–3 cm apart, and parallel to muscle fibers. A grounding electrode can be placed on another area of the body such as the abdomen, gluteus maximus anterior thigh area. Wider electrode placement will increase the amount of tissues that are emitting signals, vs. narrow spacing that results in higher specificity. It is advised to place the electrodes in an area with minimal hair and to make sure the skin is cleaned first to reduce erratic signals. Additionally, a good ionic gel or self-adhesive electrodes should be applied at each use to minimize electrode movement at the skin surface that can cause an increase in motion artifact.

When using biofeedback equipment, it is important to compare results in only the same session vs. in between sessions. It is also advised not to make in between subject recommendations or make comparison between different days in regards to PFM function. You cannot assume sEMG is isolating activity of a particular muscle since it records all the voltages leading into an electrode.[9] A contracted or shortened muscle may also be electrically silent and effect sEMG readings. Electrode placement, hormones, and vaginal secretions can also affect reproducibility of the pelvic floor signal. Secondary to the above, it is of good practice to not overly focus on the microvolt number but rather the actual correct use of the muscles during sessions.

Parks, Porter, and Malezak discovered in 1962 that the pelvic floor and external anal sphincter were activated at rest to maintain continence by comparing the pelvic floor muscles and external anal sphincter among subjects who were healthy, paraplegic, or had undergone a rectal excision.[10] Later research by Cram in 1983 that used handheld scanning electrodes in 14 other sites of the body in 104 patients led to 2 mV (microvolts) being used as the standard baseline resting value of the pelvic floor muscles.[8] More evidence-based research needs to be performed to establish pelvic floor resting norms.

Computerized data acquisition biofeedback systems are commonly used to transfer and save data for optimal clinical assessment and documenting muscle event responses over time. When assessing the pelvic floor muscles using sEMG biofeedback, observing the muscle activity for at least 1–2 minutes at rest is a great place to start. Observe if the patient knows how to relax the pelvic floor muscles actively or if general higher tone is causing an increase in resting value measurements using 2mV as a relative benchmark. Different postures such as sitting vs. standing will affect readings and should be taken into account. To measure power through quick contractions, instruct the patient in a 2-second contraction for 10 repetitions. Observe if they are able to coordinate quick contractions of the pelvic floor muscles with returning back towards resting value smoothly. You can also observe if the patient is able to maintain the intensity of each contraction by observing if the number on the screen is decreasing after a couple repetitions. For an endurance assessment, instruct the patient to contract for 10 seconds and observe how the number changes and if they are able to maintain the same level of microvolts for the whole 10 seconds. For example, in a patient with poor endurance, they may contract the muscles resulting in an increase in the number on the screen, then suddenly drop off before 10 seconds are completed. Or, you may see the patient drop off before 10 seconds but then quickly re-contract the pelvic floor muscles. When recording results, again it is imperative to not focus on numbers but rather the series of events the numbers represent. For example, rather than recording "the patient achieved a 10 mV contraction," focus on recording an event like "the patient required a 5 second delay to return to baseline value after pelvic floor muscle contraction." It is also imperative to look out for muscle substitutions patients may perform to achieve pelvic floor muscle contraction. Common mistakes patients make while trying to perform proper pelvic floor muscle contractions are breath holding, engaging gluteus maximus contractions and hip adductor muscle compensations, using toe and upper chest muscles, and bulging down on the pelvic floor, an entire opposite behavior. During biofeedback sessions, the therapist should be watching for all of these substitutions and not just be looking at the machine to decrease inaccurate assessments.

Biofeedback systems can be used at home to optimize pelvic floor retraining exercises. Using biofeedback as part of a home exercise program is great for motivating patients who may need more structured training, have poor motor and sensory awareness, or have difficulty traveling to physical therapy appointments. Units can be pre-programmed with work/rest/repetition ratios. For uptraining of pelvic floor muscles, random or blocked practice consisting of both phasic and tonic muscle contractions can be programmed into a machine. Submaximal and maximal effort contractions can also both be included into an exercise program. For downtraining of the pelvic floor muscles, patients can be asked to maintain a lower microvolt intensity while simultaneously practicing other techniques for pelvic floor relaxation such as diaphragmatic breathing and use of imagery. Both uptraining and downtraining scenarios can be advanced to functional activities that cause symptoms. For coordination training, combinations of both pelvic floor muscle contractions and pelvic floor muscle relaxation can be performed at rest and during functional activities of importance.

Biofeedback for stress urinary incontinence (SUI)

Research has shown that biofeedback can provide value to successful treatment of SUI, the involuntary loss of urine with increases in abdominal pressure, with the hopes of avoiding surgery. In a recent double-blind randomized control trial, Terlikowski *et al.* evaluated the results of treatment of SUI using transvaginal electrical stimulation and sEMG assisted biofeedback in 102 women who were pre-menopausal with SUI. The treatment group underwent two sessions per day for eight weeks. Mean urinary leakage on a pad test was significantly lower in the treatment group vs. placebo group. The treatment group also demonstrated significant improvements in muscle strength on the Oxford scale at 8 and 16 weeks, and significant improvements in quality of life.[11] Dannecker *et al.* performed a retrospective study of 390 women with SUI or mixed urinary incontinence that evaluated the short- and long-term efficacy of an intensive EMG-biofeedback-assisted pelvic floor muscle training program. EMG-biofeedback assisted pelvic floor muscle training was performed by two specially trained therapists and electric stimulation preceded pelvic floor muscle training if the pelvic floor muscle contractions were considered too weak for active training (Oxford <2). There was a statistically significant improvement in the cough test, a significant increase in the Oxford-score by 1.2 points, and self-reported improvement of incontinence symptoms was 95 short term. 2.8 years later, 71% of study participants self-reported a persisting improvement of their incontinence symptoms, showing long-term results are possible.[12] Biofeedback may be more effective for SUI in post-partum women vs. post-menopausal women. Improvements in SUI post biofeedback training has been shown to have greater improvements in post-partum women when compared to post-menopausal women in 107 women post an eight week training program, however, biofeedback training benefited both groups.[13]

Male urinary incontinence is significantly associated with urological and abdominal surgery. Biofeedback with EMG has been shown to be beneficial in improving symptoms of urinary incontinence in males with benign prostatic hypertrophy, prostate malignant neoplasm, post-prostatectomy or abdominal surgery. Twenty–thirty minute sessions of EMG biofeedback in the above male population supervised by a physical therapist twice a week showed significant improvement in both the International Consultation on Incontinence-Short Form and Incontinence Quality-of-Life Measure questionnaires. SUI was the most common type of urinary incontinence in the male population above (86.67%), followed by mixed urinary incontinence (8.33%) and urge urinary incontinence (5%).[14]

There may be debate if the addition of biofeedback training to traditional pelvic floor muscle training has any additional benefits for the treatment of SUI. A recent randomized control trial consisting of 46 women with SUI showed there was no apparent add-on effect to using biofeedback vs. traditional pelvic floor muscle strengthening in a 12-week program, however, higher quality studies may be needed on this.[15] In a systematic review, Herderschee *et al.* determined no statistical significant difference for cure rates of SUI and a small significant difference for amount of leakage episodes associated with SUI when biofeedback was added to pelvic floor muscle training. It is important to note that women who received biofeedback were less likely to report they were not improved. However, consideration needs to be taken that it is possible that women receiving biofeedback usually have more contact with the therapist which can affect outcomes.[16]

Biofeedback for urge incontinence and overactive bladder (OAB)

Many cases of urge incontinence are associated with involuntary detrusor contractions on urodynamic studies and referred to as motor urgency. Neurological deficits can also cause detrusor hyperreflexia, often referred to as a neurogenic bladder. Sensory urgency is urge incontinence in the absence of detrusor overactivity. Urge incontinence may somewhat benefit from biofeedback training, but in those with less severe detrusor overactivity.[17] Resnick *et al.* studied predictors of response to biofeedback-assisted pelvic muscle training and determined factors that mediate responses in 183 women over the age of 60 with urge urinary incontinence. Biofeedback was performed over four biweekly visits. Median urge urinary frequency decreased from 3.2/day to 1/day. Urge urinary incontinence improved by ≥50% in 55% of subjects and by 100% in 13% of subjects. Severe detrusor overactivity predicted poor response. Good response was mediated by the ability to reduce detrusor overactivity.[18] Wang *et al.* determined that electrical stimulation was superior to biofeedback assisted pelvic floor muscle training during a 12-week treatment period for urge incontinence in 103 women. However, unlike research regarding SUI, Wang *et al.* did show that biofeedback assisted pelvic floor muscle training was more effective for the treatment of urge incontinence than traditional pelvic floor muscle training alone.[19]

Dysfunctional voiding and OAB can also be a common challenge for pediatric patients. Biofeedback therapy can be an effective treatment for children with OAB and dysfunctional voiding. Significant improvement was seen in urinary tract infections (UTIs), urge incontinence, fractionated voiding, constipation, and uroflow parameters for children with dysfunctional voiding and significant improvements were seen in UTI, frequency, urge incontinence, and uroflow parameters in children with OAB in a sample of 45 children. More improvements were seen in children with dysfunctional voiding vs. OABs.[20] The addition of biofeedback therapy is an invaluable tool to help therapists retrain children's voiding habits if needed.

Many current studies have highly variable protocols for biofeedback when treating different forms of urinary incontinence, which requires further research for the future to establish standard protocols. In 2006, Glazer and Laine performed a literature review determining that biofeedback was superior to no treatment control groups, biofeedback showed mixed results to being superior to unassisted pelvic floor muscle exercises, and biofeedback was superior to oxybutynin and placebo in two studies. Biofeedback also showed mixed results when compared to vaginal cones in two studies and biofeedback and electrical stimulation showed no significant difference in benefits compared to each other.[21] Further research has continued since then and patient cases should be considered on an individual basis with what will fit their lifestyle and benefit their specific symptoms the most.

Biofeedback for colorectal pathology

Biofeedback can also be a valuable tool for patients with colorectal issues such as obstructive defecation. Ba-Bai-Ke-Re *et al.* concluded that manometric biofeedback guided pelvic floor exercises were more effective than oral polyethylene glycol therapy for obstructive defecation in 88 patients with constipation.[22] Chiarioni *et al.* found similar results in patients with chronic severe pelvic floor dyssynergia, concluding that five sessions of biofeedback were superior to continuous polyethylene glycol therapy for improvement of symptoms.[23] However, additional studies have found that biofeedback use for patients suffering from constipation is more effective for obstructed defecation vs. those with slow transit constipation. In an additional study, Chiarioni *et al.* found that five weekly sessions of biofeedback aiming to increase rectal pressure and relax pelvic floor muscles during straining, resulted in greater improvements of pelvic floor dyssynergia vs. slow transit constipation only.[24] Similarly, Battaglia *et al.* concluded that biofeedback training significantly improved constipation symptoms at three month assessments in both patients with pelvic floor dyssynergia and slow transit constipation, however, colonic transit time was not improved in slow transit constipation patients in the long term. Additionally, long-term benefits for improvement of symptoms for slow transit constipation patients were less than pelvic floor dyssynergia patients.[25] Baker *et al.* showed improvements in dyssynergic defecation and associated abdominal symptoms in 77 patients post 6–8 weeks of biofeedback training consisting of manual/verbal feedback, sEMG, exercises using a rectal catheter, rectal balloon sensory therapy, ultrasound, pelvic floor and abdominal massage, electrical stimulation, core strengthening and stretching in order to correct maladaptive dyssynergic behaviors during simulated defecation.[26] Biofeedback also shows some promising research to help improve chronic constipation and encopresis in children ages 5–16. Benninga *et al.* demonstrated that 90% of a sample of 29 pediatric patients learned proper relaxation of the external anal sphincter with significant increase in defecation frequency with decreasing encopresis after an average of five biofeedback sessions for about 35–45 minutes using an anorectal probe with an inflatable balloon. Post six weeks of training, 55% of the pediatric patients were symptoms free with maintenance at 12-month follow-up.[27]

Biofeedback for pelvic pain

Biofeedback may also offer many benefits for patients struggling with pelvic pain. Patients with pelvic pain may have point tenderness over the levator ani. Biofeedback sessions to teach pelvic floor relaxation of the levator ani may help improve symptoms. Chiarioni *et al.* compared the effectiveness of biofeedback to teach pelvic floor relaxation, electrogalvanic stimulation (EGS), or massage of levator muscles for treatment of levator ani syndrome in 157 patients over nine sessions of one of the above treatments along with psychological counseling. Patients with tenderness on rectal examination were likely to report adequate improvements from biofeedback therapy the most (87%) vs. EGS (45%) or massage (22%). Patients lacking point tenderness over the levator ani but with possible levator ani syndrome were not likely to benefit from biofeedback.[28] Vulvar vestibulitis can cause dramatic negative implications on a woman's sexual functioning. In 1995, Glazer *et al.* researched the use of EMG biofeedback with internal vaginal sensors for women with vulvar vestibulitis syndrome. Results indicated after about 16 weeks of practice, resting tension levels of the pelvic floor muscles decreased and pelvic floor muscle contractions increased. Subjective pain reports decreased about 83%. Twenty eight out of 33 patients had abstained from intercourse on average for 13 months and resumed sexual activity at the end of treatment and follow-up. Seventeen of the 33 patients reported pain free intercourse at six months follow-up.[29] Danielsson *et al.* compared biofeedback treatment using at home training programs and assessments in the office vs. topical lidocaine gel for the treatment of 46 women with vulvar vestibulitis. Post-treatment, both groups increased their pain thresholds at two vestibular sites, sexual functioning, and quality of life measurements at 12-month follow-up. However, compliance to the biofeedback program was low vs. the lidocaine treatment which may be a general challenge in using specific at home training programs. Combinations of both treatments have the potential to provide further benefits. Men specifically with chronic pelvic pain syndrome (CPPS) may benefit from biofeedback therapy to train relaxation and contraction of the pelvic floor muscles.[30] Cornel *et al.* showed improvement of pelvic pain symptoms on the Chronic Prostatitis Symptom Index (CPSI) and pelvic floor muscle tone in a sample of 31 men post biofeedback training.[31]

When treating pelvic pain patients, it is critical to compare your digital assessment to your EMG findings. If your patient presents as weak on EMG readings and cannot create high mV activity, it is the digital palpation that wins and decides the treatment plan. Patients who present with overactive pelvic floor activity should not try to increase their mV contraction ability. Their muscles present as weak because they are overactive and will not benefit from pelvic floor muscle up-training. To the contrary, it will make their pelvic pain symptoms worse. It is theorized that the EMG mV reading presents as normal or weak due to the shortening of the muscle unit, less sarcomeres within the muscle and is too tight and not of normal muscle length. Digital palpation overrules the use of biofeedback for "strengthening" for these patients. If biofeedback is required to be part of this patient's plan of care, then they need to work on downtraining.

Conclusion

Biofeedback is an effective tool and also depends upon the type of learner your patient is. Those who are visual adult learners are likely to benefit the most from biofeedback. Even those who speak a different language can benefit from biofeedback as the picture gives them the information that they may be missing. Combining biofeedback with other treatments can help optimize patient outcomes secondary to giving patients power to control their treatments. It also allows the patient to have a greater understanding of appropriate muscle sequencing during various events and positions to help decrease their pain. Biofeedback has been shown in current research studies to be an effective treatment in a variety of pelvic floor disorders. Further research is needed to help establish standardized treatment programs for certain pelvic floor disorders.

Biofeedback for erectile dysfunction

Erectile dysfunction, the inability to achieve or maintain an erection for satisfactory sexual performance, can have dramatic negative effects on a male's quality of life. Dorey *et al.* showed that three months of pelvic floor exercises and manometric biofeedback in a sample of 55 men with erectile dysfunction, showed improvements in erectile function and increase in digital anal grades and pressure vs. advice on lifestyle changes only. At six months, patients continued to improve with pelvic floor and biofeedback treatments, showing long lasting effects. Van Kampen *et al.* also showed promising results with using biofeedback assisted pelvic floor muscle exercises in a sample of 51 men with erectile dysfunction. Sessions were once a week for four months with a physical therapist consisting of pelvic floor muscle exercises enhanced by biofeedback and electrical stimulation. Of the 51 men, 47% of patients regained normal erectile function, 24% improved, 12% remained unchanged, and 18% did not complete the program. Of the 18% who did not complete the program more were considered to have psychological impotence vs. patients who completed the program. Men post-radical prostatectomy also are at high risk for developing erectile dysfunction due to intraoperative injury to neurovascular bundles. Prota *et al.* observed the effects of pelvic floor biofeedback training in men post-radical prostatectomy and its effects on recovering erectile function. Men in the treatment group began receiving pelvic floor biofeedback on post op day 15 once a week for 30 minute sessions for a total of 12 weeks by a physical therapist. Results per the International Index of Erectile Dysfunction-5, showed that the time to recover the ability to achieve an erection was significantly lower in the treatment group vs. control group. Additionally, at 12 months post op, more subjects in the treatment group were considered potent vs. the control group. Thus, early pelvic floor biofeedback muscle training post op radical prostatectomy has a significant impact on recovery of erectile dysfunction.

References

1. Ernst E and Fialka V. Ice freezes pain? A review of the clinical effectiveness of analgesic cold therapy. *J Pain Symptom Manage.* 1994;9(1):56–59.
2. Petrofsky JS and Laymon M. Heat transfer to deep tissue: the effect of body fat and heating modality. *J Med Eng Technol.* 2009;33(5): 337–348.
3. Hay-Smith EJ. Therapeutic ultrasound for postpartum perineal pain and dyspareunia. *Cochrane Database Syst Rev.* 2000(2):Cd000495.
4. Sikiru L, Shmaila H and Muhammed SA. Transcutaneous electrical nerve stimulation (TENS) in the symptomatic management of chronic prostatitis/chronic pelvic pain syndrome: A placebo-control randomized trial. *Int Braz J Urol.* 2008;34(6):708–713; discussion 714.

5. Bo K, Berghmans B, Morkved S and Kampen MV. *Evidence-Based Physical Therapy for the Pelvic Floor: Bridging Science and Clinical Practice, 2e.* London: Churchill Livingstone; 2015.
6. Morris L and Newton RA. Use of high voltage pulsed galvanic stimulation for patients with levator ani syndrome. *Phys Ther.* 1987;67(10): 1522–1525.
7. Lamina S, Hanif S and Gagarawa YS. Short wave diathermy in the symptomatic management of chronic pelvic inflammatory disease pain: A randomized controlled trial. *Physiother Res Int.* 2011;16(1): 50–56.
8. Cram JR and Kasman GS. *Introduction to Surface Electromyography.* Aspen Publishers; 1998.
9. Auchincloss CC and McLean L. The reliability of surface EMG recorded from the pelvic floor muscles. *J Neurosci Methods.* 2009;182(1):85–96.
10. Parks AG, Porter NH and Melzak J. Experimental study of the reflex mechanism controlling the muscle of the pelvic floor. *Dis Colon Rectum.* 1962;5:407–414.
11. Terlikowski R, Dobrzycka B, Kinalski M, Kuryliszyn-Moskal A and Terlikowski SJ. Transvaginal electrical stimulation with surface-EMG biofeedback in managing stress urinary incontinence in women of premenopausal age: a double-blind, placebo-controlled, randomized clinical trial. *Int Urogynecol J.* 2013;24(10):1631–1638.
12. Dannecker C, Wolf V, Raab R, Hepp H and Anthuber C. EMG-biofeedback assisted pelvic floor muscle training is an effective therapy of stress urinary or mixed incontinence: a 7-year experience with 390 patients. *Arch Gynecol Obstet.* 2005;273(2):93–97.
13. Liu J, Zeng J, Wang H, Zhou Y and Zeng C. Effect of pelvic floor muscle training with biofeedback on stress urinary incontinence in postpartum and post-menopausal women. *Zhonghua Fu Chan Ke Za Zhi.* 2014;49(10):754–757.
14. Fernandez-Cuadros ME, Nieto-Blasco J, Geanini-Yaguez A, Ciprian-Nieto D, Padilla-Fernandez B and Lorenzo-Gomez MF. Male urinary incontinence: associated risk factors and electromyography biofeedback results in quality of life. *Am J Mens Health.* 2015.
15. Hirakawa T, Suzuki S, Kato K, Gotoh M and Yoshikawa Y. Randomized controlled trial of pelvic floor muscle training with or without biofeedback for urinary incontinence. *Int Urogynecol J.* 2013;24(8): 1347–1354.

16. Herderschee R, Hay-Smith EC, Herbison GP, Roovers JP and Heineman MJ. Feedback or biofeedback to augment pelvic floor muscle training for urinary incontinence in women: shortened version of a Cochrane systematic review. *Neurourol Urodyn.* 2013;32(4):325–329.

17. Glazer HI and Laine CD. Pelvic floor muscle biofeedback in the treatment of urinary incontinence: a literature review. *Appl Psychophysiol Biofeedback.* 2006;31(3):187–201.

18. Resnick NM, Perera S, Tadic S, *et al.* What predicts and what mediates the response of urge urinary incontinence to biofeedback? *Neurourol Urodyn.* 2013;32(5):408–415.

19. Wang AC, Wang YY and Chen MC. Single-blind, randomized trial of pelvic floor muscle training, biofeedback-assisted pelvic floor muscle training, and electrical stimulation in the management of overactive bladder. *Urology.* 2004;63(1):61–66.

20. Tugtepe H, Thomas DT, Ergun R, *et al.* Comparison of biofeedback therapy in children with treatment-refractory dysfunctional voiding and overactive bladder. *Urology.* 2015;85(4):900–904.

21. Smith BE, Littlewood C and May S. An update of stabilisation exercises for low back pain: A systematic review with meta-analysis. *BMC Musculoskelet Disord.* 2014;15:416.

22. Ba-Bai-Ke-Re MM, Wen NR, Hu YL, *et al.* Biofeedback-guided pelvic floor exercise therapy for obstructive defecation: an effective alternative. *World J Gastroenterol.* 2014;20(27):9162–9169.

23. Chiarioni G, Whitehead WE, Pezza V, Morelli A and Bassotti G. Biofeedback is superior to laxatives for normal transit constipation due to pelvic floor dyssynergia. *Gastroenterology.* 2006; 130(3):657–664.

24. Chiarioni G, Salandini L and Whitehead WE. Biofeedback benefits only patients with outlet dysfunction, not patients with isolated slow transit constipation. *Gastroenterology.* 2005;129(1):86–97.

25. Battaglia E, Serra AM, Buonafede G, *et al.* Long-term study on the effects of visual biofeedback and muscle training as a therapeutic modality in pelvic floor dyssynergia and slow-transit constipation. *Dis Colon Rectum.* 2004;47(1):90–95.

26. Baker J, Eswaran S, Saad R, *et al.* Abdominal Symptoms are Common and Benefit from Biofeedback Therapy in Patients with Dyssynergic Defecation. *Clin TransGastroenterol.* 2015;6:e105.

27. Benninga MA and Buller HA, Taminiau JA. Biofeedback training in chronic constipation. *Arch Dis Child.* 1993;68(1):126–129.
28. Chiarioni G, Nardo A, Vantini I, Romito A and Whitehead WE. Biofeedback is superior to electrogalvanic stimulation and massage for treatment of levator ani syndrome. *Gastroenterology.* 2010; 138(4):1321–1329.
29. Glazer HI, Rodke G, Swencionis C, Hertz R and Young AW. Treatment of vulvar vestibulitis syndrome with electromyographic biofeedback of pelvic floor musculature. *J Reprod Med.* 1995;40(4):283–290.
30. Danielsson I, Torstensson T, Brodda-Jansen G and Bohm-Starke N. EMG biofeedback versus topical lidocaine gel: A randomized study for the treatment of women with vulvar vestibulitis. *Acta Obstet Gynecol Scand.* 2006;85(11):1360–1367.
31. Cornel EB, van Haarst EP, Schaarsberg RW and Geels J. The effect of biofeedback physical therapy in men with Chronic Pelvic Pain Syndrome Type III. *Eur Urol.* 2005;47(5):607–611.

Chapter 9

Yoga

Dustienne Miller

*Flourish Physical Therapy, Optimizing Pelvic
and Orthopedic Health, Boston, MA 02116–3635*

Yoga has been used as an adjunct treatment modality for fibromy-algia, back pain and other comorbidities associated with chronic pelvic pain (CPP). This chapter introduces practitioners to warm-ups and yoga postures used to address urological conditions associated with pain and/or weakness. Neuromuscular re-education, decreasing central sensitization, breath retraining, postural aware-ness, decreasing pain and increasing function are the goals of using yoga as an adjunct treatment for urological disorders.

Brief History of Yoga

Yoga continues to gain popularity around the world as a holistic movement therapy. In *Light on Yoga*, B. K. S. Iyengar describes the etiology of the word yoga from the Sanskrit root *yuj*, meaning to bind, join, attach, and yoke. Yoga is the union of the mind, body, and spirit. Patanjali's eight Limbs of Yoga are the corner-stones of all styles of *Hatha Yoga* taught today. The eight limbs are *yama, niyama, asana, pranayama, pratyahara, dharana, dhyana,* and *samadhi*. For the sake of brevity, the author will discuss two of the eight limbs in this chapter: *pranayama* and *asana*. Please refer to Alexandra Mispaw's chapter for a discussion on mindfulness and meditation; two valuable aspects of a yoga practice.

Efficacy of Yoga as a Movement Therapy

Currently, there are no clinical trials specifically on the use of yoga as a treatment for chronic pelvic pain (CPP). However, research has been published on the efficacy of yoga on the comorbidities associated with CPP. Clinical experience, one component of evidence-based practice as defined by the American Physical Therapy Association, has revealed yoga as a successful modality for men and women with pelvic floor dysfunction. Yoga is beneficial for dysmenorrhea,[1] anxiety,[2] fibromyalgia[2,3] irritable bowel syndrome,[4] the emotional impact of menstrual irregularities[5,6] anxiety connected with polycystic ovarian syndrome,[7] low back pain,[8–10] neurogenic bladder,[11] and urge and stress urinary incontinence (SUI).[12]

Clinical evidence supports that yoga can:

- Increase strength, flexibility, vigor, acceptance, relaxation, compassion, and heart rate variability
- Decrease pain, fatigue, emotional distress, anxiety, depression, stress, and resting heart rate
- Improve cardiovascular function, sleep patterns, quality of life, self-awareness, mindfulness, and digestive function

In the clinical setting, physical therapists and other healthcare providers incorporate yoga postures and breathing techniques during treatment as a form of neuromuscular reeducation. Postural reeducation can be practiced in Mountain Pose. Twists are helpful for releasing restrictions through the abdominal and pelvic cavities and can be used as visceral mobilization. The concepts of central sensitization, graded motor imagery, and graded tolerance can all be incorporated into practice by introducing pain-free, successful movement. Prescribed warm-ups and *asana* enhance core stability, increase flexibility and encourage proper sequencing of muscle firing patterns.

Pranayama

Iyengar describes *pranayama* as "extension of breath and its control".[13] *Pranayama* includes inhalation, exhalation, and breath retention. Breathing is a critical component of rehabilitation for pelvic floor dysfunction. Clinicians describe a piston-like relationship between the diaphragm and pelvic floor.[14,15] *Pranayama*, or conscious breathing can enhance this relationship, especially when there are muscular holding patterns in the pelvic girdle. On inhalation, the pelvic floor and diaphragm lengthen caudally. On exhalation, the pelvic floor and diaphragm shorten cranially.[16] Practitioners instruct students to use the breath in coordination with the pelvic floor muscles (PFMs) to obtain optimal stability and continence. Visualizations can be helpful for encouraging downtraining or uptraining of the PFM. The concept of coordinating the breath with the PFM contraction is explored in Table 1.

Pelvic organ prolapse (POP) and urinary/fecal incontinence are often caused by lack of tonic support and muscular strength of the pelvic floor and surrounding pelvic girdle musculature.[17] Optimal pelvic floor support from adequate strength, core

Table 1.   Breath Cues — Visualizations for the Breath and PFM

Landmark	Inhale	Exhale
Abdomen	Softens, expands away from midline	Comes back into center
Mid/lower ribcage	Expands away from midline	Comes back into center
Ischial tuberosities	Separate, soften, float away from each other	Come back into center
Coccyx	Lengthens away from pubic bone	Floats back toward pubic bone
Pelvic floor muscles	Lengthen out and down/open like pinball flippers	Come back in toward body

stability and neuromuscular control allows for continence and organ support. For optimal core stability, there must be coordination and strength of all components of the deep core musculature—PFM, transverse abdominals, multifidi, and diaphragm.[19] The "Soda Pop Can Model of Postural Control", conceptualized by Mary Massery illustrates how the core canister of support of a soda can is maintained by optimal pressures, thus maintaining the stability of the structure. Loss of support at the top tab of the soda can, (i.e. tracheotomy) affects postural control. Loss of support at the front (i.e. diastasis recti) or bottom (i.e. POP or incontinence) affects postural control and core stability.[18] This concept emphasizes the importance of breath retraining within rehabilitation.

Benefits of *Pranayama*

Pranayama gives your patient a strategy to decrease sympathetic nervous system over-activity and increase the parasympathetic response. According to Diane Lee, two common areas of rigidity of movement/holding patterns include lateral and posterior-lateral expansion of the ribcage with inhalation.[19] Mindful *pranayama* encourages the student to explore diaphragmatic breathing without gripping in the chest and ribcage. Practicing side bending postures like *Ardha Chandrasana* combine the lateral expansion of the rib cage during inhalation with lengthening quadratus lumborum and latissimus dorsi.

Examples of *Pranayama*

Dirgha is the Three-Part Breath.

1. Inhale into the belly.
2. Allow the breath to expand the ribcage.
3. Send the breath caudally as the collarbones to float up.

When this rhythm is established you can layer on the *Ujjayi* Breath (explained below). After trying this for 10 breath cycles, stop and recognize any new sensations or softening in the body. Practice a 10 breath cycle in the morning, just before bed, and any other time during the day when pain or stress increases.

Ujjayi is the Ocean Breath. This breath should sound similar to the signature sound of the Star Wars villain Darth Vader. Perform this breath with any warm-up or *asana*.

1. Raise one hand in front of the mouth and pretend to fog a mirror with an inhalation and exhalation.
2. Recreate the same action at the back of the throat, but now with the mouth closed.

Nadi Shodhana is known as the Alternate-Nostril Breath/ Channel-Purifying Breath.

1. Shaping the right hand in Vishnu mudra (4th and 5th fingers bend halfway), close off the right nostril gently with the thumb.
2. Exhale, then inhale through the left nostril.
3. Switch the nostril plug to the left side with the ring finger.
4. Exhale and inhale through the right nostril.
5. Switch the nostril plug to the right side using the thumb.
6. Continue for 10 breaths or as desired.

Keep the breath smooth, long, meditative and gentle to balance the hemispheres of the brain, soothe the nervous system, and quiet the mind. The easy way to remember the sequence is like the song "Old MacDonald Had a Farm".... E(xhale), I(nhale), E, I, O(ther nostril).

Letting Go Breath is a quick check in to access instant awareness to the areas in the body that habitually hold tension.

1. Inhale through the nose.
2. Gentle exhale with an audible sigh through the mouth.

Bandhas

Moola Bandha is a commonly practiced bandha (lock) in which the perineal body is lifted cranially.[20] For men and women with overactivity of the pelvic floor and abdominal muscles, it is advised to only use *moola bandha* for awareness of the PFM.

For men and women who desire to strengthen the PFM, *band-has* are appropriate to practice, as long as the contraction does not become an overuse holding pattern. When strengthening the PFM, it is important to address the entire core's ability to activate and sequence appropriately rather than just isolating *moola bandha*. This includes hip/glute strengthening, dynamic balance training, functional training and coordination of the PFM with different tasks, PNF, and other rehab techniques.

Connecting the Breath with the Pelvic Floor

Sadly, some clients still report being told by a medical professional to "just relax", "have a glass of wine", or "stop holding your pelvic floor tight". If only it were that easy! Visualization using bony landmarks can help ground the ethereal idea of "releasing the pelvic floor". We can offer breath cue visualizations to encourage optimal breathing patterns and relaxation of the PFM. If the client desires to strengthen the pelvic floor, accentuate the PFM concentric contraction during exhalation and coordinate this movement with a contraction of the transverse abdominals.

Asana

Asana, or physical postures, are the most widely known aspect of yoga. Prior to performing *asana*, warm-ups are an ideal way to introduce movement. Gentle and slow movements combined with conscious breathing, act to warm up muscles, lubricate joints, and direct the focus of the student inward to the mind–body–spirit connection. The author recommends starting a yoga practice by warming up each direction of the spine: flexion/extension, right/left side bend, and right/left rotation. There are numerous warm-ups to choose from. For the sake of brevity, the author chose three warm-ups for this chapter.

Warm-ups

Cat/Cow

Start in table top position on hands and knees with hands directly under shoulders and knees directly under hips.

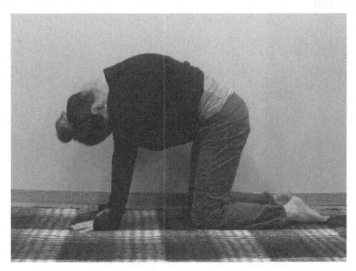

1. Inhale, prepare for movement.
2. Exhale, pull the belly button up towards the spine into lumbar flexion, looking toward the navel.

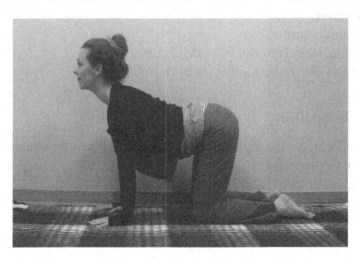

3. Inhale, send the ischial tuberosities and coccyx up toward the ceiling, arching the back and softening the chest toward the floor.
4. Repeat for 5–10 breaths.

Wag the Tail

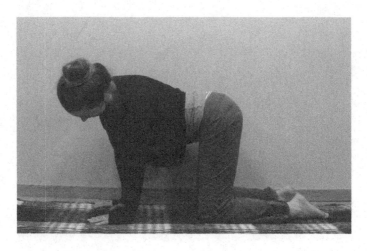

1. Inhale to prepare.
2. Exhale, draw the right shoulder towards the right hip. The movement of hiking the hip towards the shoulder will create a C curve in the spine. If desired, bring the right ear to the right shoulder.
3. Inhale to center.
4. Exhale, switch to the left side C curve.
5. Repeat alternating sides for 5–10 breaths.

Thoracic Rotation

1. Inhale, bend the right elbow, keep the left elbow straight and look to the left.
2. Exhale, untwist, and come back to table top.
3. Inhale, bend the left elbow, keep the right elbow straight and look to the right.

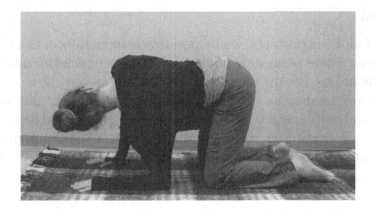

4. Exhale, untwist, and come back to table top.
5. Repeat alternating sides for five breaths.

Rock Backs

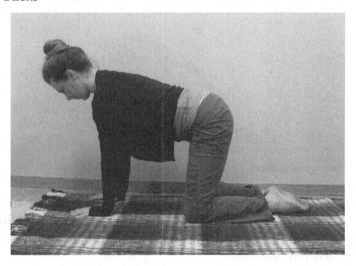

1. Start in table top with feet together and knees apart.
2. Inhale, shift pelvis back keeping the spine neutral, bending only at the hip crease.
3. Exhale, pull torso back to the starting point, keeping the hands planted and pulling back with the core.
4. Rock back for five breaths.

Asana

The following postures can be performed separately or as part of a series. There are several postures that are beneficial for urological disorders. For the sake of brevity, the author has chosen a few postures to discuss in depth. Not every client has the same physical profile, so it is best to evaluate each patient and prescribe postures according to the patient's musculoskeletal needs. Instruct your patients to move consciously in and out of the postures and use props such as pillows, blankets, and cushions, to make the postures as comfortable as possible.

Child's Pose (*Garbhasana*)

Child's Pose is a popular yoga posture and often prescribed in physical therapy to increase lumbopelvic flexibility.

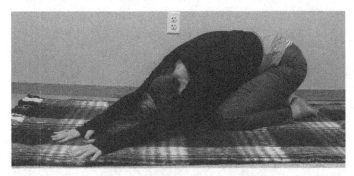

Instructions: Start in table top. Bring the feet together and rock back so the buttocks are on the heels and the chest is resting on the thighs. Feel the lateral and posterior–lateral expansion of the rib cage with inhalation.

Modifications: Place a blanket under the thighs (for limited knee ROM, rolled towel under the top of the ankle (for limited ankle ROM), blanket at the hip crease to increase the hip angle (open the knees more for anterior hip impingement), forehead on stacked fists or a bolster.

Benefits: Child's Pose increases lumbopelvic flexibility and calms the sympathetic nervous system. Some students feel an additional stretch in the anterior thigh and ankle. As the student releases into the posture, the abdomen softens towards the floor. For students with gastrointestinal issues, this can be a helpful posture for releasing gas. This posture offers an opportunity for imagery of the PFM from the access point of the ischial tuberosities. Bringing attention to the sitz bones, imagine drawing a circle around the ischial tuberosity, softening the tissue around the attachment sites of the hamstrings, adductors, and sacrotuberous ligament.

Variation: To increase flexibility of the latissimus dorsi and improve respiration: Walk the hands, arms, and shoulders to the right. Feel the left rib cage expanding laterally on inhalation. Exhale, allowing the body to settle towards the floor. Hold for 5–10 breaths and repeat on the other side.

Prescription: Choose this posture for your patients with constipation, overactive bladder (OAB), interstitial cystitis/painful bladder syndrome (IC/PBS), and dysmenorrhea.

Special note: Transform child's pose into a restorative posture. Place a bolster between the inner thighs, reaching the spine long as the student lays forward. Hug the arms around the front end of the bolster.

Sphinx (*Bhujangasana*)

Sphinx is a gentle spinal extension posture that can be used alone or as a preparation for a deeper back bend, i.e.: cobra or upward facing dog.

Instructions: Start prone. Press the top of the feet and pubic bone into the ground as the arms reach forward. The elbows are directly underneath the shoulders, forearms connecting with the ground, and palms and fingers press into the mat. Keep the cervical spine neutral, reaching out through the top of the head and out through the feet.

Modifications: Place a pillow under the abdomen if the stretch is too intense in the lumbar spine or abdomen; rest the chest on a pillow.

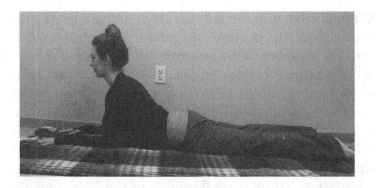

Benefits: Shoulder stabilization; myofascial release of the abdomen; increases tissue excursion post-abdominal surgery; strengthens back musculature; lengthening of the abdominal wall without overstretching the anterior hip capsule.

Variations: Squeeze a block between hands for isometric shoulder internal rotation; pull a resistance band outward for shoulder external rotation.

Contraindications: Spondylolisthesis, 2nd/3rd trimester, recent abdominal surgery.

Precautions: Limited trunk extension ROM; pain that increases with extension i.e.: spinal stenosis, sacroiliac dysfunction; active flare of bladder or abdominal pain/menstrual pain/endometriosis.

Prescription: Choose this posture for your patients with OAB, IC/PBS, dysmenorrhea and constipation.

Supine Twist (*Supta Matsyendrasana*)

Supine Twist is a gentle twist that can be used alone or as a preparation for a deeper twist i.e.: revolved triangle pose. Twists are an effective myofascial release for the abdomen and helpful for digestive issues, including constipation.

Instructions: Start supine with knees bent, feet on the ground, arms out to the side, and palms facing the ceiling. Inhale. Exhale, bringing the knees to the left. Stay for 3–5 breaths, encouraging lateral expansion of the rib cage as the abdomen rises to the

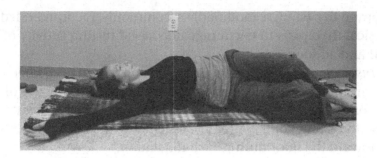

ceiling during inhalation. To switch knees to the right, engage the abdominals on the exhalation. Stay for 3–5 breaths.

Modifications: Place a block or pillow under the knee to decrease the shear at the sacroiliac joint; place a block or pillow between the knees to decrease hip internal rotation of the top leg; recline on pillow during the second and third trimester.

Benefits: Myofascial release of the abdomen and chest wall; increases tissue excursion post-abdominal surgery.

Contraindication: Recent abdominal surgery.

Precautions: Lumbopelvic pain that increases with spinal rotation.

Prescription: Choose this posture for your patients with coccydynia, OAB, IC/PBS, and constipation.

Happy Baby (*Ananda Balasana*)

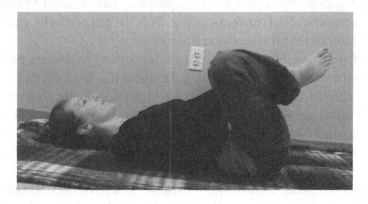

Happy Baby (shown modified) is commonly recommended by physical therapists to encourage decreased resting activity of the PFM and adductors.

Instructions: Start supine in hip flexion/abduction, knee flexion, and ankle dorsiflexion. Hands can hold the outside of the feet, or wherever the student can reach. Keep sacrum heavy and spine long. Stay for 3–5 breaths, visualizing the coccyx lengthening toward the floor during each inhalation.

Modifications: Grab the inside of the ankles and open the knees wider; place a strap over the arches, practice one side at a time with the other leg extended on the ground.

Benefits: Increases flexibility of the posterior thighs and adductors; releases lumbar spine; calms the sympathetic nervous system; releases PFM.

Variations: Pelvic floor drop: resist the knees as they press into flexion/abduction/external rotation.

Contraindication: $2^{nd}/3^{rd}$ trimester of pregnancy.

Precautions: Lumbopelvic or hip pain that increases with hip flexion.

Prescription: Choose this posture for your patients with coccyx pain, OAB, and vulvar pain.

Downward Facing Dog (*Adho Mukha Shvanasana*)

Downward Facing Dog is an inversion pose that allows quieting of the sympathetic nervous system, enabling the student to experience a moment of introspection. This is particularly valuable when coupled with conscious breathing.

Instructions: Start in table top. Send the sitz bones back to where the wall meets the ceiling, keeping the back straight. The knees should be bent if there are restrictions in the hamstrings and lumbar spine. Feet can walk back until the first sensation of stretch is achieved. While breathing in this posture, visualize the tailbone reaching toward the ceiling during inhalation, allowing the pelvic floor muscles to release.

Modifications: If the patient experiences wrist pain, modify by placing the forearms on the ground (Dolphin Pose). For those

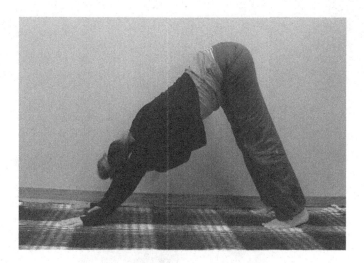

unable to transfer to the ground, or during pregnancy, the palms can be on a wall with a flat back and hip angle at 90°.

Benefits: Increases flexibility and retrains muscular holding patterns; elongates the myofascial planes of the plantar fascia, calves, hamstrings, sacrotuberous ligaments, PFMs; builds core strength; elongates the spine.

Variations: Pedal the feet, alternating knee flexion ("walking the dog"), lift one leg up in the air ("downdog split").

Contraindication: Uncontrolled high or low blood pressure; shoulder/wrist injury.

Precautions: Acute pudendal neuropathic pain that is irritated with hip flexion; restrictions in the hamstrings and low back (bend knees to modify).

Prescription: Choose this posture for your patients with coccyx pain, prolapse, and vulvar pain.

Note: Downward Facing Dog can become a restorative posture by resting the chest and hip crease on a plinth or bed.

Half Moon (*Ardha Chandrasana*)

Half Moon offers an opportunity to build postural awareness and strength in a standing pose while lengthening the side body.

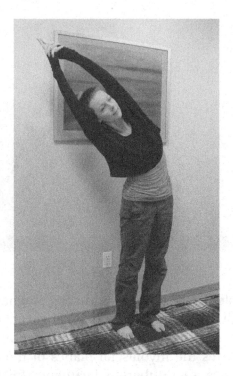

Instructions: Start in Mountain Pose with feet hip distance apart, rib cage over pelvis, scapula down the back, neck long. Inhale the arms up and overhead. Exhale and bring the hands into a steeple position. Inhale, reach long and over to the right with the upper body while the pelvis and legs stay heavy and grounded. Press down through the left foot to further elongate the tensor fasciae latae. Exhale, reaching out to come back to neutral. Repeat on the other side. Add an additional pelvic shear to the side away from the direction of the arms for an additional lateral stretch.

Modifications: For limited shoulder range of motion or pain, use a strap or keep the arms down with the strap behind the back. If the pull is too intense at the lateral hip, focus on the side bending the trunk.

Benefits: Myofascial release of the lateral line; increases rib mobility and diaphragmatic excursion, increases flexibility of the latissimus dorsi and quadratus lumborum.

Variations: Allow the pelvis to shift to the opposite side of where the hands and arms are reaching, encouraging further elongation of lateral line.

Precautions: Watch alignment for those with sacral torsions: use the verbal cue "Imagine you are between two planes of glass"; spasm of the quadratus lumborum.

Prescription: Choose this posture for your patients with coccyx pain, constipation, and pudendal neuralgia.

Warrior 1 (*Virabhadrasana*)

Warrior 1 is a grounding standing posture that can be performed with the hand on the wall or a chair for balance.

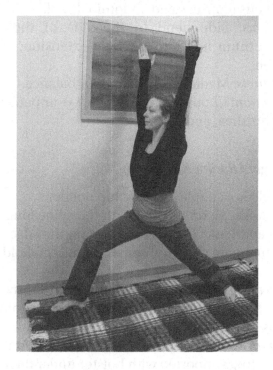

Instructions: Start in Mountain Pose. Squat halfway, keeping the spine long and bending only from the hip crease. Send the right leg back, coming into a split stance. The left knee bends, but not forward over the toes. Keep the left knee in line with the second toe. Traditionally, the right leg turns out slightly, but the author teaches this posture first with a parallel back leg for knee sensitivities and pelvic floor dysfunction irritated by external rotation of the hip. If the student tolerates the back leg in external rotation, encourage both anterior superior iliac spines (ASIS) to remain facing the front of the mat. Inhale the arms up, palms facing each other. Hold for five breaths.

Modifications: Turn back leg parallel to avoid adverse tension at the medial aspect of the knee; widen the base of support as needed for balance; hands on hips for shoulder discomfort.

Benefits: Strengthens the lower extremity; increases proprioception; improves balance; lengthens anterior thigh and adductors; lengthens iliopsoas and abdominal wall.

Variations: Side bend to the side of the knee that is forward; sternum lifts into thoracic extension; vary degree of knee flexion.

Precautions: Medial knee pain; poor balance.

Prescription: Choose this posture for your patients with stress UI, dysmenorrhea, and IC/PBS.

Bound Angle (*Badha Konasana*)

Bound Angle is a simple and safe hip opener.

Instructions: Sit on the mat with the spine long, feet together and knees apart. Ask the patient to sit on the edge of a blanket if unable to maintain a neutral spine. Hands can hold the ankles or feet.

Modifications: Sit on a pillow or bolster to accommodate for tight hamstrings, weak spinal erectors and/or hip restrictions; recline this posture if the patient experiences vulvar pain (*supta badha konasana*); if the patient experiences sacral pain, modify with supine frog supported with bolster under the knees.

Benefits: Adductor and PFM release.

Variations: Seated pelvic clock; spinal flexion/extension/rotation/SB.

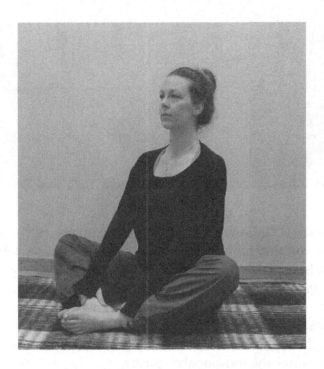

Precautions: Sacral pain; pain with sitting (vulvar and pudendal neuropathic pain); limited hip external rotation; limited hip flexion.

Prescription: Choose this posture for your patients with IC/PBS, vulvar pain, and dysmenorrhea.

Restorative Fish (*Matsyasana*)

Restorative Fish opens the chest and encourages ease with breathing.

Instructions: Place the bolster lengthwise on the mat. Bring the ischial tuberosities to the edge of the bolster and on the ground. Lie back over the bolster and open the arms out to the side with the palms to the ceiling. Legs can be bent, out straight, in half lotus, up the wall or in *badha konasana* (feet together,

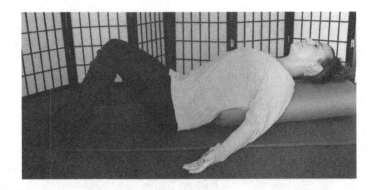

knees apart). Optional leg strap at the thighs can encourage releasing of the hips. Additional blankets can be added for warmth. Stay in this position for 3–10 minutes.

Modifications: Towel under the head for those with forward head posture; blocks/blankets under the knees if legs are in *badha konasana*; bolster under knees if legs out straight.

Benefits: Opens the chest wall, calms the sympathetic nervous system, relaxes the lumbopelvic girdle.

Precautions: For sensitivity with lumbar extension, take a blanket perpendicular to the mat and place it at the mid-thoracic spine instead of a bolster and support with the bolster under the knees.

Prescription: Choose this posture for your patients with constipation, dysmenorrhea, OAB, and IC/PBS.

Restorative Goddess

Restorative Goddess allows for deep relaxation, hip opening, and calming of the sympathetic nervous system.

Instructions: Place the bolster lengthwise on the mat. Support the head of the bolster with a block, blanket, or bolster. Bring the ischial tuberosities to the edge of the bolster and still on the ground. Lay back over the bolster and open the arms out to the side, palms to the ceiling. Legs can be out straight, in half lotus, or in *badha konasana* (feet together, knees apart). With the legs in *badha*

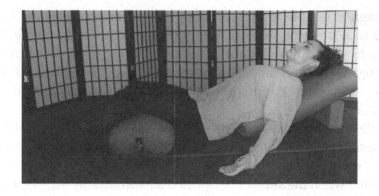

konasana, a strap can be placed at the sacrum, over the anterior thigh, and looping over the dorsal aspect of the foot for further support. Additional blankets can be added for warmth. Stay here for 3–10 minutes.

Modifications: Towel under the head for those with forward head posture; blocks/blankets under the knees if legs are in Badha Konasana; bolster under knees if legs are out straight.

Benefits: Opens the chest wall, calms the sympathetic nervous system, and relaxes the lumbopelvic girdle.

Contraindications: Coccyx pain; sacroiliac pain.

Precautions: If sensitive to lumbar extension or coccyx pain, create a ramp at the bottom of the bolster to decrease the angle and soften the floor to accommodate for structures in the posterior pelvic girdle.

Prescription: Choose this posture for your patients with vulvar pain, dysmenorrhea, IC/PBS, and OAB.

Savasana

Traditionally, yoga practice ends with Corpse Pose, or Savasana (also spelled *Shavasana*). In *Savasana*, the patient experiences a physical letting go (muscles relaxing, physiological quieting) and the deeper mental space of being aware of what is going on around you while simultaneously being present to the self. If the student is unable to creating the time/space for Savasana at the end of a practice session, the author recommends taking 5–10 breaths focusing on grounding down through the sitz bones if sitting, or through the feet if standing. This gives the body–mind–spirit a moment to integrate the changes that occurred during practice.

Research performed by Sharma *et al.* on the benefits of Savasana demonstrated a decrease in systolic blood pressure, diastolic blood pressure, pulse rate, respiratory rate, and rate pressure product when the subject performed *Savasana* daily for 10 minutes for four weeks. It suggests that a person practicing Savasana can successfully reduce the physiological effects of stress.[21]

Postural Awareness and Prolapse

One benefit of a consistent yoga practice is improved postural awareness in daily activities. Body mechanics and maintaining good spinal health is important not only for CPP disorders but also for urological disorders with supportive dysfunction. Research by Sapsford *et al.* showed an increase in resting activity of the PFM in the asymptomatic (no UI) group, which correlated with increased lumbar lordosis. PFM activity influences bladder inhibition and provides support to the pelvic organs. Over time, adopting a non-slumped posture may protect against POP and UI, as the PFM are less active in the slumped posture. Therefore, the perfect storm of decreased lumbar lordosis, decreased PFM activity, and decreased support of the pelvic organs may increase the risk for UI and POP.[22]

Unweighting the pelvic floor a few times during the day can be helpful for POP. Practicing supported bridge with a bolster or block under the sacrum is restorative to the pelvic girdle. PFM contractions can be practiced in this posture. Maintaining good bowel habits (stool consistency, not straining, etc.), strengthening the lumbopelvic girdle, avoiding valsalva, and coordinating the breath/core/pelvic floor with lifting will help prevent the POP from getting worse.

Conclusions

I hope this chapter serves as a launching off point to learn more about yoga and other available movement therapies. When prescribing postures, please be mindful of the possibility of trauma. Remind the patient often that they must listen to their body to guide what feels appropriate for them and never to try to push through the pain.

References

1. Rakhshaee Z. Effect of three yoga poses (cobra, cat and fish poses) in women with primary dysmenorrhea: a randomized clinical trial. *J Pediatr Adolesc Gynecol.* 2011;24(4):192–196.
2. Katzman MA, Vermani M, Gerbarg PL, *et al.* A multicomponent yoga-based, breath intervention program as an adjunctive treatment in patients suffering from generalized anxiety disorder with or without comorbidities. *Int J Yoga.* 2012;5(1):57–65.
3. Curtis K, Osadchuk A and Katz J. An eight-week yoga intervention is associated with improvements in pain, psychological functioning and mindfulness, and changes in cortisol levels in women with fibromyalgia. *J Pain Res.* 2011;4:189–201.
4. Evans S, Cousins L, Tsao JC, Sternlieb B and Zeltzer LK. Protocol for a randomized controlled study of Iyengar yoga for youth with irritable bowel syndrome. *Trials.* 2011;12:15.
5. Rani K, Tiwari S, Singh U, Agrawal G, Ghildiyal A and Srivastava N. Impact of Yoga Nidra on psychological general wellbeing in patients with menstrual irregularities: A randomized controlled trial. *Int J Yoga.* 2011;4(1):20–25.
6. Rani K, Tiwari S, Singh U, Singh I and Srivastava N. Yoga Nidra as a complementary treatment of anxiety and depressive symptoms in patients with menstrual disorder. *Int J Yoga.* 2012;5(1):52–56.
7. Nidhi R, Padmalatha V, Nagarathna R and Amritanshu R. Effect of holistic yoga program on anxiety symptoms in adolescent girls with polycystic ovarian syndrome: A randomized control trial. *Int J Yoga.* 2012;5(2):112–117.
8. Saper RB, Sherman KJ, Cullum-Dugan D, Davis RB, Phillips RS and Culpepper L. Yoga for chronic low back pain in a predominantly minority population: a pilot randomized controlled trial. *Altern Ther Health Med.* 2009;15(6):18–27.

9. Tilbrook HE, Cox H, Hewitt CE, *et al.* Yoga for chronic low back pain: a randomized trial. *Ann Intern Med.* 2011;155(9):569–578.
10. Patil NJ, Nagaratna R, Garner C, Raghuram NV and Crisan R. Effect of integrated Yoga on neurogenic bladder dysfunction in patients with multiple sclerosis-A prospective observational case series. *Complement Ther Med.* 2012;20(6):424–430.
11. Tekur P, Nagarathna R, Chametcha S, Hankey A and Nagendra HR. A comprehensive yoga programs improves pain, anxiety and depression in chronic low back pain patients more than exercise: an RCT. *Complement Ther Med.* 2012;20(3):107–118.
12. Huang AJ, Jenny HE, Chesney MA, Schembri M and Subak LL. A group-based yoga therapy intervention for urinary incontinence in women: a pilot randomized trial. *Female Pelvic Med Reconstr Surg.* 2014;20(3):147–154.
13. Iyengar BKS. *Light on Yoga: Yoga Dipika.* Schocken; 1995.
14. Sapsford RR, Richardson CA, Maher CF and Hodges PW. Pelvic floor muscle activity in different sitting postures in continent and incontinent women. *Arch Phys Med Rehabil.* 2008;89(9):1741–1747.
15. Julie Wiebe, Physical Therapist | Educator, Advocate, Clinician. 2015. Available on: http://www.juliewiebept.com/.
16. Talasz H, Kremser C, Kofler M, Kalchschmid E, Lechleitner M and Rudisch A. Phase-locked parallel movement of diaphragm and pelvic floor during breathing and coughing-a dynamic MRI investigation in healthy females. *Int Urogynecol J.* 2011;22(1):61–68.
17. Sapsford R. Rehabilitation of pelvic floor muscles utilizing trunk stabilization. *Man Ther.* 2004;9(1):3–12.
18. Massery M. The linda crane memorial lecture: The Patient Puzzle: Piecing it Together. *Cardiopulm Phys Ther J.* 2009;20(2): 19–27.
19. Lee DG. *The Pelvic Girdle: An integration of clinical expertise and research, 4e.* Churchill Livingstone; 2010.
20. Buddhananda S. *Moola Bandha: The Master Key.* Yoga Pubns Trust; 1998.
21. Sharma G, Mahajan KK and Sharma L. Shavasana-Relaxtion technique to combat stress. *J Bodyw Mov Ther.* 2007;11:173–180.
22. Sapsford RR and Hodges PW. The effect of abdominal and pelvic floor muscle activation on urine flow in women. *Int Urogynecol J.* 2012;23(9):1225–1230.

Chapter 10

Osteopathy for Urologic and Pelvic Health

Daniel Lopez

Osteopathy New York, PC New York, NY 10003

Osteopathic medicine deals with normalizing and optimizing the health of the patient. A large component of this is by making sure there are no anatomical derangements affecting its ability to function properly. This chapter provides a brief introduction to osteopathy and how it may help in assessing and treating pelvic problems.

Introduction

"We look at the body in health as meaning perfection and harmony, not in one part, but in the whole." Andrew Taylor Still, M.D., D.O.[1]

In the United States, the osteopathic profession produces fully licensed physicians with full practice rights in all 50 states. Most osteopathic physicians, or D.O.s, currently practice medicine alongside M.D.s as equals. One thing that distinguishes osteopathic doctors from their M.D. counterparts is training in osteopathic manipulative medicine (OMM). This gives osteopathic physicians an added dimension in assessing and treating their patients. This chapter will focus on that.

Historically, osteopathic medicine dates back to the 1800's. In 1874, Andrew Taylor Still, M.D., DO, founded osteopathic medicine. He looked for a "better way" after losing many family members to meningitis. This was a time when there were no antibiotics, and the standard medical practices often caused more harm than good such as blood-letting.[2]

Dr. Still followed principles that he observed in nature and applied them to the human body for health. Dr. Still realized that optimal health requires all the tissues and cells of the body to function together in harmonious motion. He reasoned that disease could take hold in the body whenever there were anatomical deviations from normal, no matter how slight they may be. Anatomical deviations are not necessarily the cause of disease, but can produce the environments where disease can take place. This is evident when he writes "Osteopathy is based on the perfection of Nature's work. When all parts of the human body are in line we have health. When they are not the effect is disease."[3]

Studying living, dynamic anatomy, he learned how the body worked as a functional unit. In his book *Philosophy of Osteopathy*, he writes, "You begin with anatomy, and you end with anatomy, a knowledge of anatomy is all you want or need ..." Keeping this in mind, he would work to find "health" by restoring the anatomical deviations back to normal with his hands. Dr. Still used this style of medicine to treat many infectious diseases, including meningitis, dysentery, whooping cough, influenza, measles, mumps, and rubella. As a profession, osteopathic physicians successfully treated many patients using osteopathic manipulative treatment (OMT) during the Spanish flu pandemic of 1918–1919 that killed 40,000,000 worldwide and 650,000 in the United States.[4]

Dr. Still felt the body contained the resources for healing and fighting infections. The osteopathic physician's job was to facilitate healing by removing any obstruction, no matter how slight, that could be impeding the body from functioning optimally. This would bring about health. Currently, OMT is mostly used to treat musculoskeletal aches and pains anywhere in the body more than infectious diseases as was originally done.

Over time, the osteopathic profession laid out principles which would become the foundation for osteopathic medicine:

- There is a relationship between the body's structure and function
- The body is a unit, with the health of the patient being a combination of mind, body and spirit
- The body has an innate ability to self-regulate and self-heal
- Rational treatment is based on the above three principles

These are consistent with many of Dr. Still's original teachings, and an osteopathic physician works with these same principles today. Dr. Still did not teach techniques but left osteopathic medicine open ended for osteopathic physicians as science and knowledge grew. Osteopathy is a philosophy on health. Since Dr. Still's time, osteopathic physicians have added to the body of work. Although there are standard techniques taught in osteopathic medical school, as long as any technique applied by the osteopathic physician follows the principles above, it falls under the category of OMT.

Many bodywork modalities today have their origins in the osteopathic profession including myofascial work, strain counterstrain techniques, craniosacral therapy, visceral manipulation, and more. Presently, osteopathic physicians that practice OMT represent a small minority of the osteopathic profession. Those who practice OMT still work with osteopathic principles to treat their patient's problems. In order to treat urologic or pelvic problems, osteopathic physicians still use their hands to feel for subtle anatomical abnormalities throughout the whole body to assess how they may be causing the patient's problem, use their understanding of anatomy, and restore normal health as much as the body will allow.

Although more research is needed in regard to OMT and treating pelvic problems, there are some small studies showing promise for larger studies. Some studies have shown efficacy in treating primary dysmenorrhea and pain during pregnancy.[5–9] Anecdotally, osteopathic physicians have reported success with helping patients with urinary issues, pelvic pain, bladder dysfunctions, and more. Studies are still lacking to show efficacy of OMT with their respective issues.

Assessment

An osteopathic structural exam will include an assessment of the whole body prior to performing any treatment. Because the focus is on urologic and pelvic issues, it is assumed that a full body assessment would be performed prior to keying in on these areas. Osteopathic physicians palpate for changes that indicate a deviation from normal anatomy to abnormal. These changes can be found on any structure in the body, not just the musculoskeletal system. They may include tenderness, asymmetry, restricted motion and tissue texture changes. This chapter will focus solely on the potential anatomical causes of pelvic and urologic issues. In this chapter, it will not be possible to cover every anatomical structure that may be assessed and potentially treated. It is assumed that other causes have already been considered and worked up.

There are multiple ways that osteopathic physicians may use to assess for these changes. For this reason, the focus will be on the anatomy that may be important factors in contributing to their respective problems with potential reasons. No patients are exactly the same and each will have different factors contributing to their problem. The job of the osteopathic physician is to understand how the dysfunctions throughout the patient's body are creating their specific symptoms.

For issues with the pelvis, some important bony structures to evaluate for dysfunctions are the innominate bones, sacrum, coccyx, and corresponding sympathetic spinal segments.

Through palpation, the joints are evaluated for motion along different planes to assess for restriction and signs of dysfunction. Anteriorly, the innominate bones articulate with each other at the pubic symphysis, a cartilaginous joint. Motion at the pubic symphysis can be complex. It is thought that the pubic bones move about a transverse axis corresponding to ilial motion. The pubic bones may also become sheared. This means that one pubic bone may have shifted superiorly, inferiorly, anterior, or posterior compared to the other along with their respective innominate.[10]

Dysfunctions at the pubic bone have reportedly been a cause for bladder dysfunction due to the bladder lying directly posterior to the pubic symphysis, the endopelvic fascia, and the pubovesical ligament.[11] With pubic dysfunction, fascial tension on the urogenital diaphragm can affect genitourinary (GU) function. Pubic bone dysfunctions should be evaluated with pelvic floor problems and pain due to the attachments of pelvic floor muscles such as the pubococcygeus and puborectalis, muscles of that form the levator ani group. Some osteopathic physicians have reported pubic symphysis dysfunctions as being capable of producing urinary frequency and may mimic symptoms of urinary tract infections (UTIs) in women due to its influence on the bladder. Osteopathic physicians may test for motion at the pubic symphysis by evaluating the position of specific landmarks on pubic bones relative to each other and testing their motion by gliding them along different planes of motion.

Posteriorly, the innominate bones articulate with the sacrum at the sacroiliac joints. The innominate bones can be viewed as extensions of the lower extremities during walking and will rotate anteriorly and posterior during gait. In addition, the anterior superior iliac spines (ASIS) can inflare or outflare. This means that they may rotate toward or away from the midline about a vertical axis. They may become sheared as described above where one innominate bone shifts superiorly or inferiorly in respect to the other.[10] A common way of evaluating this motion is with the patient lying supine. Using a handhold over the ASIS, the osteopathic physician can then test how the innominate bones move along different planes of motion.

Motion to assess for dysfunctions is also evaluated at the ischial tuberosities. Ischial tuberosity dysfunctions are often considered with pelvic floor problems including pain, incontinence, and more. They are often evaluated by palpating and moving them laterally and superiorly. A tender and tenser ischial tuberosity will indicate a dysfunction here. Dysfunctions at the ischial tuberosities can have significant impact to the pudendal nerve when involvement is suspected. Arising from the sacral plexus, three nerve roots exit located immediately above the upper border of the sacrotuberous ligament and ischiococcygeus muscle. The pudendal nerve proper forms just proximal to the sacrospinous ligament. Structural abnormalities here can compress or influence the proper function of the pudendal nerve. The pudendal nerve innervates motor function to many pelvic floor muscles and sensory to the penis in males and clitoris in females.

Motion at the sacrum is often evaluated. Sacral motion is highly complex and there are varying models describing its motion. Its ability to move is influenced by its L5 articulation above it and the innominate bones laterally. There are also ligamentous attachments such as the sacrotuberous and sacrospinous ligaments that will influence the movement of the sacrum. In females, the uterosacral ligaments may have an effect on the sacrum or vice versa. In general, the sacrum can move about transverse, oblique and vertical axes. Sacral dysfunctions are considered highly important because of their ability to influence the parasympathetic nervous system exiting at the levels of S2-4 and pudendal nerve arising from the sacral plexus that influence many structures in the pelvis.[10] Also, the sacrum has dural attachments at the levels of S2-4. The sacrum may be evaluated prone or supine and motion may be evaluated along all of its planes of motion.

At the apex of the sacrum, it articulates with the coccyx. The coccyx may be palpated both externally and internally to evaluate its range of motion and position. Its position may be driven by the position of the sacrum and the muscles attached to it including pubococcygeus, ischiococcygeus, and lower fibers of the gluteus maximus muscles. The filum terminale links the coccyx to the dural membranes in the sacrum. The coccygeal plexus gives rise to the coccygeal nerve that has sensory innervation over the coccyx. Dysfunctions in the coccyx can have an effect on the stability of the pelvic floor. With coccydynia, a trauma will often move the coccyx. It can be highly important in these cases to assess how all the structures of the pelvis and pelvic floor may have been affected as well and help restore normal motion and function the coccyx.

Other structures to consider are the autonomic corresponding segments of the spine or sacrum to influence the autonomic nervous system. There may be viscerosomato reflexes or somatovisceral reflexes. A viscerosomatic reflex refers to a dysfunction or irritation producing reflex structural changes over the musculoskeletal system. A somatovisceral reflex refers to a problem over the musculoskeletal system that will reflexively affect an organ's ability to be healthy. An example of a somatovisceral reflex may be a sacral dysfunction affecting the parasympathetic innervation to the organs of the pelvis. An example of a viscerosomatic reflex may be kidney stones having an effect on the vertebrae corresponding to the sympathetic innervation. Interestingly, this will change as a stone moves along its course. As part of an acute process, the vertebrae over the region affected may also feel warm compared to the surrounding areas.[10]

Pelvic organ problems may produce sacral dysfunctions because of the effect they may have on the parasympathetic nervous system. The corresponding sympathetic innervation should be considered as well. For example, the parasympathetic innervation for the bladder arises from the sacrum and the sympathetic innervation for the bladder arises from approximately T10-L1.[10] These may be important regions to assess and treat when dealing with bladder problems to help balance the autonomic nervous system.

The organs themselves may be evaluated for their position and fascial tension on them. The organs are suspended in the abdomen and pelvis by a series of fascial and ligamentous attachments. Abdominal and pelvic organ positioning and their corresponding fascia can have a strong effect on the overall musculoskeletal system. For example, the bladder may be isolated and assessed over the pubic bones. From there, the tension on the ureters may be assessed. Retroperitoneal organs like the sigmoid colon and kidneys may be palpated and influenced by an anterior and posterior handhold.

One last structure in this chapter that may be of importance to assess is the psoas muscle. The psoas muscle arises from L1-5, crosses the sacroiliac joint and femoral coal joint and attaches to the lesser trochanter of the femur. Lying just anterior to the transverse processes of the lumbar vertebrae over the lumbar plexus, it has several nerves that pierce it or course right next to it. The genitofemoral nerve pierces directly through the muscle belly and the lateral cutaneous nerve of the thigh and the femoral nerve that come out from its lateral border. The kidneys also often lie just over the psoas muscle and may move along its plane when they move from the correct positioning.

Each patient will be evaluated according to their respective problem. The osteopathic physician will reason their way anatomically based on their findings as to why the patient will be experiencing their set of symptoms. Potential problem areas would be assessed and then treated with OMT if appropriate. In some cases, they may refer out to another specialist if necessary.

Treatment

There is often a misunderstanding with OMT and what it is. OMT is simply the application of osteopathic principles to the patient. It is not defined by a set of techniques as was explained earlier but can be open-ended. During osteopathic medical training, there are standard techniques that osteopathic students learn. We will discuss those although they are not all encompassing and OMT specialists may use more advanced techniques. With any technique, it is important for the osteopathic physician understand the limitations of the technique, indications, and contraindications to know when to apply or not apply them. Below is a brief review of some standard techniques:

High-velocity/Low-amplitude (HVLA)

HVLA is the technique that is the most known. These techniques involve isolating a dysfunctional joint and quickly thrusting within its anatomical barrier. The thrust is rapid but the motion very slight. This is what is meant by "high-velocity/low-amplitude". Often, this technique is followed by an audible "pop" although that is not necessary for the success of the treatment. This technique is commonly used and can produce rapid improvement in mobility and pain relief. However, it also is limited to joint dysfunctions, may contribute to joint instability, and is not appropriate all of the time.[12]

Muscle Energy (ME)

ME is defined as "a form of OMT in which the patient's muscles are actively used on request, from a precisely controlled position, is a specific direction, and against a distinctly executed counterforce." FOM 682 ME technique was credited to Fred Mitchell Sr. where he developed it in the 1940's and 1950's. It uses the concept of post-isometric relaxation to treat myofascial pain. ME technique is contraindicated in acute injuries and any situation where the patient cannot cooperate among others. Applied appropriately, ME has few complications and can have good results.[13]

Myofascial Release (MFR)

MFR is a system of diagnosis and treatment that goes back to the origins of osteopathy. MFR utilizes continues monitoring through palpatory feedback to achieve a release of myofascial tissues. Tissues can be loaded with constant directional force until a tissue is released and motion is restored. Additionally, tissues can be positioned in a direction where ease is identified toward the least resistance until a release is noted and tissue movement is achieved. A combination of the above can also be accomplished. There are no absolute contraindications with this technique but relative contraindications exist based on regional or local problems such as open wounds or recent surgery. MFR techniques have few complications and can have good results when performed by a skilled osteopathic physician.[14]

Strain–counterstrain technique

This is a technique developed by Lawrence H. Jones, D.O. in 1955. It is often referred to simply as counterstrain. It positions the patient in a position away from their restrictive barrier in a position of maximum comfort for the patient. This is done to treat tender points throughout the body. When an optimal position is achieved, the tenderness of the tender point disappears. The treatment process once the optimal position is achieved until the release is finished takes about 90 seconds and may be palpated as a pulsation by the practitioner. This technique is indicated whenever a tender point is palpated. Contraindications involve fractures but otherwise, there are few contraindications. The treatments are tolerated well and rarely produce post-treatment reactions.[15]

Osteopathy in the Cranial Field (OCF)

OCF applies osteopathic principles to the skull and its effects to the rest of the body. It has its roots with William Garner Sutherland, D.O. with the concept going back as far as 1899. It is based on applying subtle therapeutic forces to release anatomical dysfunctions noted in the skull. Dr. Sutherland described a model which was named the primary respiratory mechanism (PRM). This model has five components:

1. The inherent rhythmic motion of the brain and spinal cord.
2. Fluctuation of the Cerebrospinal Fluid.
3. Mobility of intracranial and intraspinal membranes.

4. Articular mobility of the cranial bones.
5. Involuntary mobility of the sacrum between the ilia.

This concept may be applied for pelvic floor dysfunctions because of the link between the head and sacrum via dural membranes. The treatment is meant to influence the nervous system as well and may be used to treat the sacrum. As a result, it can have an effect on the pelvis. OCF techniques have few contraindications such as skull fractures. OCF treatments have few complications and are generally tolerated well.[16]

Conclusions

Finally to conclude the chapter, I would like to share a story. This was one of my first experiences seeing what osteopathy could achieve. This is the story of a woman in her early 50's named Gloria. For about 10 years, Gloria had suffered with a problem with urinary frequency. Gloria had to urinate sometimes over 30 times per day. This problem had been getting worse and was so bad that her whole life revolved around this problem. She was afraid of going on long drives, of going to the movies, or any other activities where she may not have immediate access to a bathroom.

Unfortunately, Gloria had been to many specialists and tried every medication that was available for her problem at the time. Nothing had worked. This caused her to feel more and more despondent as nothing worked and her internist began to run out of ideas. Finally, he admitted to her that he did not know what else to do. The last options that he could think of was to refer her to a psychiatrist or to have her enroll in a trial surgery. None of which were great options.

I was in my first year of training when I watched my mentor perform osteopathy on Gloria. She was visiting from another state when she came to see him. He analyzed her whole body and found that there were some anatomical dysfunctions in the bony pelvis. He found some significant findings in her skull. Lastly, he felt what he described as a "twist" in her bladder that was irritating a ureter. Gently using his hands, he helped her body resolve the issues that it had not been able to by itself.

Once he was done, he mentioned that the anatomy felt correct and her body would continue to make the changes it could. Gloria flew home after that visit. Immediately, she felt improvement. Over the next couple weeks, her symptoms continued to improve until they went away completely. After this, she moved on with her life as if nothing had ever happened and her symptoms over a decade later have never returned. I know the story of Gloria very well. Gloria is my mother.

Like my mentor, I have had the good fortune of being able to use osteopathy to help patients that have come through my office with problems from pelvic pain to incomplete voiding after prostate surgery. Osteopathy is a great non-invasive, conservative approach for many problems including problems related to the pelvis.

References

1. Still AT. *The Philosophy and Mechanical Principles of Osteopathy.* Kirksville, MO: Osteopathic Enterprise; 1986.
2. Trowbridge C. *Andrew Taylor Still, 1828–1917.* Kirksville, MO: Truman State University Press; 1991.
3. Still AT. *Osteopathy, Research and Practice (HardPress Classics).* HardPress Publishing; 2012.
4. Gevitz N. *The DOs: Osteopathic Medicine in America.* Johns Hopkins University Press; 2004.
5. Molins-Cubero S, Rodriguez-Blanco C, Oliva-Pascual-Vaca A, Heredia-Rizo AM, Bosca-Gandia JJ and Ricard F. Changes in pain perception after pelvis manipulation in women with primary dysmenorrhea: a randomized controlled trial. *Pain Med.* 2014; 15(9):1455–1463.
6. Holtzman DA, Petrocco-Napuli KL and Burke JR. Prospective case series on the effects of lumbosacral manipulation on dysmenorrhea. *J Manipulative Physiol Ther.* 2008;31(3):237–246.

7. Boesler D, Warner M, Alpers A, Finnerty EP and Kilmore MA. Efficacy of high-velocity low-amplitude manipulative technique in subjects with low-back pain during menstrual cramping. *J Am Osteopath Assoc.* 1993;93(2):203–208, 213–204.
8. Schwerla F, Wirthwein P, Rutz M and Resch KL. Osteopathic treatment in patients with primary dysmenorrhoea: A randomised controlled trial. *Int J Osteopath Med.* 2014;17(4):222–231.
9. Hensel KL, Buchanan S, Brown SK, Rodriguez M and Cruser d A. Pregnancy research on osteopathic manipulation optimizing treatment effects: the PROMOTE study. *Am J Obstet Gynecol.* 2015;212(1): 108.e101–109.
10. Heinking KP and Kappler RE. *Pelvis and Sacrum in Foundations of osteopathic medicine.* Philadelphia: Wolters Kluwer Health/Lippincott Williams & Wilkins; 2011.
11. Herschorn S. Female pelvic floor anatomy: the pelvic floor, supporting structures, and pelvic organs. *Rev Urol.* 2004;6(Suppl 5):S2–S10.
12. Hohner C. *Thrust (High Velocity/Low Amplitude) Approach; "The Pop in Foundations of osteopathic medicine.* Philadelphia: Wolters Kluwer Health/Lippincott Williams & Wilkins; 2011.
13. Ehrenfeucter WC. *Muscle Energy Approach in Foundations of osteopathic medicine.* Philadelphia: Wolters Kluwer Health/Lippincott Williams & Wilkins; 2011.
14. O'Connell J. *Myofascial Release Approach in Foundations of osteopathic medicine.* Philadelphia: Wolters Kluwer Health/Lippincott Williams & Wilkins; 2011.
15. Glover JC and Rennie PR. *Strain and counterstrain approach in Foundations of osteopathic medicine.* Philadelphia: Wolters Kluwer Health/Lippincott Williams & Wilkins; 2011.
16. King H. *Osteopathy in the Cranial Field in Foundations of osteopathic medicine.* 728–748 ed. Philadelphia: Wolters Kluwer Health/Lippincott Williams & Wilkins; 2011.

Chapter 11

Cognitive Behavioral Therapy

Alexandra Milspaw

Institute for Women in Pain, Bethlehem, PA 18018

Cognitive behavioral therapy has been used in modern medicine to treat a myriad of psychological disorders ranging from anxiety to addiction. This practice is a form of psychotherapy that focuses on changing the thought process and behavior of the patient. Health professionals work with the patient to develop techniques of rational thought with two main branches. These are problem focused and action oriented. As research progresses, scientific research has begun to utilize these skills in other clinical settings. In the urological setting, the use of cognitive behavioral therapy can have profound effects in clinical applications. This chapter will outline the use of mindfulness and cognitive behavioral therapy brain training to change the outcomes of chronic pelvic pain (CPP), an umbrella of urological disorders.

Helping the Brain Change "Painful" Habits

Chronic pelvic pain (CPP) often involves a myriad of psychological diagnoses, including, but not limited to anxiety, depression and post-traumatic stress disorder (PTSD). Research demonstrates that these diagnoses are able to be described not only by chemical imbalances in the brain, but also by physiological changes in brain structures. These same brain structures that change and transform with trauma and anxiety are also involved with the perception of nociception, thereby contributing to one's experience of physical and psychological pain. Cognitive Behavioral Therapy (CBT), Mindfulness-Based Stress Reduction (MBSR) and hypnosis have been shown to change how the brain responds to stimuli, including nociception, thoughts, and emotion. The following chapter reviews the research behind how these techniques, especially when used together, can help break the brain's habitual patterns of response and consequently decrease the experience of physical, psychological, and emotional pain. The chapter ends with a description of applicable activities and exercises that utilize the CBT and MBSR techniques.

Multidisciplinary and Integrative Approaches for the Treatment of CPP

Research on multidisciplinary approaches to CPP is rising to the surface of awareness all over the world.[1] One study from Sweden specifically looked at the longevity of the effect of pain-related multidisciplinary rehabilitation by examining the number of sickness absences from work.[2] The study was a 10-year follow up, which consisted of 214 participants suffering from chronic back pain.[2] The treatments participants received included behavior-oriented physical therapy (aerobic training, pool training, relaxation techniques, body awareness therapy, and tailored physical therapy programs), CBT (activity planning, goal setting, problem solving, applied relaxation, cognitive coping techniques, activity pacing, how to break vicious circles, assertion training and the role of significant others) and a combination of the two treatments, which the researchers labeled behavioral medicine rehabilitation (p. 1728).[2] The longitudinal data indicated that multidisciplinary rehabilitation was most successful in helping pain patients return to work as well as decrease the amount of sickness absence (p. 1733).[2]

Research on multidisciplinary interventions has also been reviewed for women specifically diagnosed with vestibulodynia. Sadownik *et al.* completed a qualitative retrospective study on 19 women who participated in a program that included education, medical management, pelvic floor physiotherapy, and mindfulness-based CBT delivered over 12–16 weeks (p. 1088). The impact of the multidisciplinary program was summarized by five major themes: "increased knowledge, gained tools/skills, perceived improved mood/psychological well-being, a sense of validation and support, and an enhanced sense of empowerment (p. 1090)."[3] The researchers go on to state that the analysis of the data found "significant improvements in psychological health, sexual health and sexual pain immediately after and at four months after discharge" from the multidisciplinary program (p. 1092).[3]

As this chapter continues to demonstrate, CPP consists of a multitude of triggers on both the physical and psychological levels. This complex problem demands an equally complex set of interventions that must be catered to the individual's needs. These interventions are summarized below.

Pain and the "Fight, Flight, or Freeze" Response

Is it fear-related pain or pain-related fear? That is the main question discussed in the book, *Pain-related fear*, by Johan *et al.* Vlaeyen *et al.*'s book is based on the most recent evidence-based research specifically focused on the parasympathetic response of the nervous system. When someone experiences pain, this triggers the emotional reaction of fear.[4] Fear triggers our brain to produce chemicals that make it more difficult for us to relax.[4] In fact, mere emotions and thoughts (both conscious and unconscious) can trigger this chemical reaction placing the nervous system in the "fight, flight, or freeze", or parasympathetic, mode.[4] When the body goes into this mode, it is an evolutionary protective response, as if there were a dangerous lion in the room.[4] As discussed earlier in this chapter, this parasympathetic mode causes muscle spasm, increased heart rate, dilated pupils, shallow breathing and other autonomic nervous system responses, such as dry mouth, slower immune response and inhibited digestion.[4] The brain then seeks more feedback from the body to know more about what's happening, increasing the sensitivity in the nervous system.[4] Our brain "turns the volume up" on our nervous system.[4] This means that our physical sensations increase and consequently we feel more pain. In other words, when it comes to pain, the more we fear it, the more we feel it. This cycle is represented in the Fear-Avoidance Model shown in Figure 1.

The fear-avoidance model was studied in relation to low back pain (LBP) by researchers Anna Dawson, Philip Schluter, Paul Hodges, Simon Stewart, and Catherine Turner. Using a sample of 2,164 working nurses and midwives with LBP, Dawson *et al.* examined the relationship between fear of movement, pain catastrophizing and passive coping and staying home from work. They found that fear of movement increased the likelihood of the participants staying home from work (p. 1522).[5]

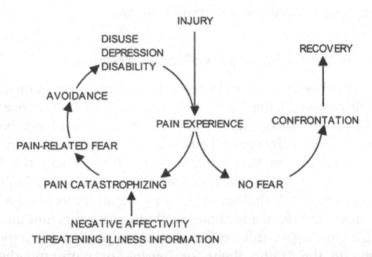

Figure 1:   An outline of Fear-Avoidance Model of Chronic Pain from Chapter 1 of *Pain-Related Fear: Exposure-Based Treatment of Chronic Pain*, by Vlaeyen J, Morley S, Linton SJ, Boersma K, and de Jong J, IASP Press, Seattle, Copyright 2012. This figure has been reproduced with permission of the International Association for the Study of Pain (IASP).

The authors also found gender differences. While the presence of fear of movement resulted in an increased sick leave in both men and women, men had "significantly increased odds of LBP-sick leave compared with women (p. 1520)".[5] However, only 8% of their sample were men (p. 1520).[5] The researchers also found that pain catastrophizing does predict fear of movement, but it does not directly relate to distal factors, such as disability and work absence (p. 1522).[5] Interestingly, the study reports that "active coping had no protective effect on LBP-sick leave," but this study did not go into exploring what those active coping skills were (p. 1522).[5] In other words, while the participants reported taking active roles in coping with their back pain, this did not seem to affect how much sick leave they took from work. The researches recommend further research into addressing active coping responses to pain that address confrontational behaviors that have a protective effect on LBP and associated sick leave.[5] This chapter will attempt to address some active coping skills that have been shown to help with chronic pain disorders.

When someone experiences pain for a prolonged period of time, this often leads to fears not only related to the concern of what is causing the pain, but also fear of participating in certain activities, such as walking or going to work or even spending time with friends.[1,4] Fear can literally paralyze someone. This is why the "fight or flight" phase is more clearly described as the "fight, flight, or freeze" phase of the nervous system.[1] Similar to what happens with a deer in the headlights, when the body is consumed with fear it freezes. Eventually, if this fear lasts for a long time it can turn into a vicious cycle, aiding in the development and maintenance of the chronic pain disorder.[4] Over time there are physiological changes that take place that aid in the increase of neurochemical generators being sent through the nervous system with a decreased amount of neurochemical inhibitors to outweigh the signals.[4] Consequently, while fear plays a major role in the continuation of chronic pain, there are other important variables and factors playing into this process on a neurobiological level.

Nevertheless, the variable of pain-related fear must be addressed in the treatment of chronic pain.[4] CBT is one of the most highly recommended and effective modalities to treat fear related to chronic pain.[4] CBT is discussed later in this chapter.

Fear of pain also influences sexual arousal and sexual functioning.[6] In a research review by Dewitte *et al.*, the authors discuss the role fear plays in causing physiological reactions, including vaginal dryness and pelvic floor hypertonicity, citing over 36 research articles (p. 251). While Dewitte *et al.* recognized that "pain is, however, a multidimensional experience that needs to be addressed in all its dimensions, including biomedical as well as psychosocial aspects," (p. 251) they performed this research review to analyze the specific role fear plays in the influence of sexual pain. They concluded, "the anticipation of pain is expected to install hypervigilance to painful sexual stimuli and to diminish attention for sexually exciting stimuli, resulting in impaired genital and subjective sexual arousal (p. 251)."[6] When looking at the sexual response cycle, "pain-related fear may impact on several of these phases (p. 252)."[6] Addressing pain-related fears and the perception of pain is important in the context of understanding and treating chronic pelvic and sexual pain. CBT, Education, and MBSR techniques address these variables of fear and perception.

Consequences of PTSD

PTSD is when our body stays in the parasympathetic mode due to trauma in our life.[7] Trauma consists of physical, emotional, psychological, or social traumas.[7] Sometimes, we experience a physical trauma we don't mind too much, such as injuries resulting from athletic activity or play. We can also experience trauma that we do not want, such as car accidents, abuse, and surgery. Our bodies can also experience trauma from persistent stress in our life stemming from work, family, finances and other life events.[7] PTSD adds to chronic pain because it keeps our body in the "fight or flight" mode, which maintains the nervous system to operate on a "high volume" level of functioning.[7] Consequently, a smaller stimulus can equal a larger reaction from the nervous system, often experienced as a greater amount of pain.[8]

When the body is in the parasympathetic state, the protective response of the nervous system, physiological changes take place in the brain, particularly with the amygdala and hippocampus.[1,4,9] The hippocampus is one of the main memory chips in the brain and is strongly affected by the chemical activity of the amygdala.[4] When someone experiences trauma, the hippocampus shrinks in size, which can result in either gaps in memory or the opposite, exaggerated clips of memory that can come back in the form of flashbacks.[4] In the context of how the brain perceives incoming signals from peripheral nerves, if the hippocampus and amygdala have been affected or are currently in a fight-or-flight state, the brain will perceive these signals as being more dangerous and therefore has a stronger reaction to those signals.[4]

Synaptic activity in the brain also changes in response to trauma.[1] The synapse is the space between which the neural connections in the brain talk to each other.[1] In a normal healthy synapse, there is a balanced chemical regulation within the synapse.[10,11] In a traumatized brain, there are either too few or too many neurotransmitters being sent across that synaptic space, resulting behaviorally in either dissociated states or hyper-aroused states.[10,11] As discussed above, the stronger the reaction, the higher the pain level is experienced. Thus, the literature supports the fact that if someone has a history of trauma, their brain may have a stronger reaction to the physiological signals being sent up through the nervous system due to the deregulation of the synaptic activity, amygdala and hippocampus.[10,11]

Several studies have documented the substantial burden of PTSD on individual health and general functioning.[7,10–12] The World Health Organization's Global Burden of Disease analysis reported that PTSD was responsible for nearly 3.5 million years of healthy life lost worldwide in 2004, including over 2.5 million in women.[12] Hidalgo and Davidson demonstrated evidence for increased lifetime physical problems and negative health behavior in veterans with PTSD, sexually assaulted women, and those exposed to traumatic events in childhood. Thus, PTSD plays a major role in millions of women's lives and is consequently a critical factor to look at when discussing the causes of central sensitization in the nervous system.

Pain catastrophizing

In discussing the neurobiology of pain and trauma, it is important to discuss the role of pain catastrophizing. The word "catastrophizing" implies that the patient is consciously choosing to exaggerate or characterize their pain as awful, horrible, and unbearable.[13] While research has shown that the act of catastrophizing pain increases the experience of pain and cortical responses to pain, [13,14] this has not been discussed within the context of the patient's history of trauma, the effect this has on the neurobiology and neural response in the brain, or the patient's knowledge about their pain disorder — all of which, as discussed earlier, affects their pain level. The study from Graceley *et al.* demonstrated that the act of catastrophizing increased neural responses to pain. According to the research discussed earlier in this chapter, it has been demonstrated that higher neural activity is associated with higher levels of pain irrespective of what causes that higher activity. In Graceley *et al.*'s study of 29 subjects with fibromyalgia, the researchers utilized functional MRI scans to view neural activity during a pain testing session after they evaluated for the level of depression, catastrophizing and clinical pain (p. 837). The researchers found that catastrophizing was significantly and positively associated with higher neural activation and reported clinical pain, independent of self-report of depressive symptoms.[13]

David Seminowicz and Karen Davis also performed a similar study, using functional MRI scans to observe participants' brain activity during a pain simulation activity. However, their study participants were categorized as healthy individuals, rather than chronic pain patients.[14] In their study of 22 participants, they found an increase in cortical regions associated with affective, attention and motor aspects of pain.[14] These were the same regions discussed in Graceley *et al.*'s (2004) study. Both studies conclude in their discussion that pain catastrophizing can aid in the progression to or persistence of chronic pain.[13,14] Thus, whether the participant has a history of chronic pain or not, pain catastrophizing increases neural activity and the experience of pain.[13,14] This confirms that the perception of the inflicted pain affects the brain's response to those incoming signals, as had been discussed in Moseley's research earlier. However, neither article discussed the participants' past history of trauma, genetic predisposition, and knowledge about how pain is processed in the brain — all of which could be additional causes to the increase in neural activation and experience of pain.[1]

Psychological treatments that help manage pain catastrophizing on a conscious level will be discussed later in this chapter. Nevertheless, it is important to take into consideration all of the unconscious, biological changes that occur in the brain out of the patient's control that affect the neural responses to pain, including the level of knowledge of their pain disorder, their history of trauma, and any genetic predisposition to chronic pain disorders, depression, and anxiety.

Psychological Treatment for CPP

The experience of living incessantly with CPP takes a huge toll on women's self-esteem, self-worth, and overall mental, emotional and spiritual wellness. "CPP is a longstanding condition and women with it are at greater risk of low self-esteem, depression or anxiety, low marital satisfaction and sexual dysfunction and somatic symptoms."[15] Chronic pain and depression are two of the most common health problems that medical and other health providers encounter, and depression is a particularly frequent comorbid diagnosis in chronic pain.[16] Furthermore, research shows that CPP patients suffering from depression also demonstrate enhanced anxiety.[9]

When psychological distress, such as depression and anxiety, is present, there is a direct effect on both pain and continued functioning.[17] In a study of 327 patients, who experienced major lower extremity trauma, researchers from Johns Hopkins University completed a longitudinal study analyzing the relationship among pain, psychological distress, and physical function (p. 1349).[17] "Greater levels of both depressed and anxious mood lead to decreasing levels of function and participation at subsequent time periods both early and late in the recovery period after injury (p. 1353)."[17]

Consequently, it is important to address this widespread problem with a widespread set of tools, techniques, and interventions that can target as many of the layers as possible. One of these important interventions includes psychophysiological therapy. "Psychophysiological therapy includes counseling and relaxation therapy, a stress-management program, and biofeedback techniques."[15] Mindfulness-based cognitive therapy involves all four of these techniques and is shown to significantly decrease anxiety and depressive symptoms.[18] In past research, physiotherapy, such as mindfulness-related techniques, has been significantly effective in improving psychomotoric function, working capacity and decreasing pain.[19]

In summary, there is a strong mind–body connection that cannot and should not be ignored when treating any chronic illness or chronic pain disorder.[20] New research coming out of the University of Rochester headed by neurobiologist David Felten is exploring a new, hybrid field of study now known as "psychoneuroimmunology (p. 4)."[21] Felten's research "has documented ways in which the brain sends signals to the immune system" and thereby "controlling their immune systems (pp. 3–4)."[22] When it comes to the healing processes and healing capabilities of the body, the mind must be intimately involved.

Cognitive Behavioral Therapy

When something like chronic pain cannot be seen it is often hard to believe it exists. The uncertainty in the minds of physicians and patients alike about the mental or physiological causes of pain produces stigmatizing reactions in others, which makes it difficult for one to talk openly about their experience.[23] Communication skills are critical within the practices of CBT, MBSR, and other self-care techniques.[18] Patients need communication skills in order to encourage the maintenance of relationships in their social, familial, and personal lives.[24] The more social support, particularly from the spouse, that the patient has, the greater their overall well-being.[24]

Cognitive-behavioral therapeutic interventions help guide clients in examining the relationship between their symptom-based distress, their thinking at such times and the motions linked with those thoughts and their behavioral responses to their particular thinking style (e.g. illness vs. wellness focused).[4] A study of 172 patients with depression only, pain only, and both depression and pain, looked at sentence completion exercises to explore the cognitive bias toward health.[25] The findings from this study "suggest that the combination of pain and depression, rather than being in pain in itself, is associated with a cognitive bias towards negative-health cognitive content".[25] Dianne Wilson *et al.* also found a link between language and the pain experience in their meta-analysis of 66 articles that examined the role of attention on pain descriptors in persistent pain patients. Thus, specific cognitive interventions are specifically needed when treating the comorbidity of pain and depression. "Cognitive strategies aimed at increasing self-efficacy as well as controlling catastrophization and hypervigilance will contribute to the reduction of pain and improvement in sexual functioning (p. 145)."[26]

CBT, the most-studied psychological treatment in chronic pain, can improve coping skills and promote improved functioning, including sexual functioning.[27] "A behavioral strategy that is a basic component of any pain[27] management program is the practice of relaxation (p. 145)."[26] CBT includes progressive relaxation, diaphragmatic breathing and setting and working toward behavioral goals.[18] One purpose of CBT within the realm of CPP is stress and pain control.[28] CBT has been shown to be effective in helping women with CPP reduce muscle contraction in the pelvic floor, reduce rumination on catastrophic thoughts about their pain, and empower them to exercise self-care techniques that reduce their stress and pain.[28]

CBT instructs the patients to challenge their automatic negative thoughts. It also asks them to replace those negative thoughts with new thoughts that feel better. If patients do not know or understand what is going on with their pain and symptoms, it is difficult for them to challenge the catastrophic thoughts. Here is where knowledge and understanding of their pain, symptoms and diagnosis are helpful.

Knowledge is power

Steege highlights in his CPP textbook that "the first step in treatment is a meeting with the patient, and, ideally, at least one family member, for the purpose of education (p. 11)." The provision of pain knowledge to patients is an effective evidence-based treatment tool.[1,29] Patients who get their questions answered will have increased satisfaction and better coping strategies, including less anxiety.[29] Patients can understand far more than most health professionals realize.[30] Moseley showed that patients and therapists can understand the neurophysiology of pain, but professionals usually underestimate the ability of patients to understand. Integrated knowledge of all pelvic organs and other systems, including musculoskeletal, neurological and psychiatric systems is the first step in effectively managing, treating, and empowering patients suffering from CPP.[15] Continuing with the idea of mind–body connections comes the understanding that the more patients understand about their bodies and about their pain, the more they are able to visualize the steps to manage and treat their symptoms; again, this leads to improved self-care efforts and thus easing pelvic pain symptoms.[20] Vlaeyen *et al.*'s Fear-Avoidance Model includes negative affectivity and threatening illness information as significant contributors to pain catastrophizing, which leads to pain-related fear, avoidance, hypervigilance, depression and disability, and ultimately a higher pain experience (p. 18). Consequently, non-threatening, valid and accurate information on the physical condition is important in the treatment of chronic pain conditions.[20] Patients who receive education on the neurophysiology of pain experience changes in regard to pain beliefs, changes in regard to attitudes, improved cognition, improved physical performance, increased pain thresholds and improved outcomes from therapeutic exercise.[4,31,32] Moseley utilizes metaphors and stories in his explanation of pain to patients as a way to help them conceptualize the neurophysiology of pain, which he finds effective in his practice. The content of the neurophysiological education includes the following: neurophysiology of pain, nociception and nociceptive pathways, neurons, synapses, action potential, spinal inhibition and facilitation, peripheral sensitization, central sensitization, and the plasticity of the nervous system.[33] Finally, psychoeducation has been demonstrated to reduce shame and embarrassment in response to some CPP symptoms, such as persistent genital arousal disorder.[34]

Transform the Brain to Create New Habits

Hypnosis and MBSR

The context of signals being sent to the brain affects the pain it evokes.[35] In other words, the mind's focus during noxious stimuli can affect how much pain the person experiences because it alters the perception of that stimuli. This is one of the reasons why hypnosis and MBSR aid in the reduction of chronic pain symptoms.

Hypnosis has been shown to decrease neural activity in the same regions that mediate the pain response.[36] Marie Faymonville and her research team examined the neural mechanisms of antinociceptive effects of hypnosis, which they report having used to produce analgesia during surgical interventions in previous studies (p. 1257). Faymonville *et al.* reviewed positron emission tomography (PET) data and magnetic resonance imaging (MRI) data on 30 healthy volunteers during pain stimulations of thermal stimuli. The researchers discuss specific criteria they utilized to ensure the level of hypnosis, including verbal and motor sluggishness, eye movements, heart and respiratory rates, and intense muscle relaxation (p. 1262).[36] The researchers made a point to note that the hypnosis "was directed toward reducing pain perception" (p. 1264). Faymonville *et al.* conclude that hypnosis intervention served to decrease cortical activity and therefore successfully reduce noxious perception and unpleasantness (p. 1266).

MBSR is the approach utilized by researchers Segal *et al.* in their book "Mindfulness-based cognitive therapy for depression." Practicing mindfulness aids in the reduction of rumination,[18] which is a significant predictor of chronic pain-related disability.[37] By practicing mindfulness, individuals can begin to notice and redirect their ruminating thoughts. Mindfulness trainer, Eckhart Tolle explains, "Such transformation is the work of mindfulness itself, brought about by paying attention in highly specific ways to the entire landscape, inner and outer, of one's experiences, including intense emotions. One might call this the path to the embodiment of emotional intelligence"[38] (p. viii). Mindfulness is the complete awareness and attention on the present moment without judgment or an attempt to change anything.[18] "When we are able to be in the present moment, we become more awake in our lives, more aware of each moment, more aware of the choices open to us," such as negative cognitive connections between behavior and emotion (p. 48).[18]

Clinical studies have shown the effectiveness of mindfulness meditation reducing pain-related fear, depressive symptoms and anxiety in women with chronic pain disorders. A study from researchers in the United Kingdom examined mindfulness in people with chronic low back pain who were attending a multidisciplinary pain management program (p. 645).[39] The researchers defined mindfulness as "moment-to-moment attention and observation of external and internal stimuli (e.g. thoughts, feelings, bodily sensations) in a non-judgmental and non-reactive way"[39] (p. 644). Participants completed a baseline questionnaire and another at a three-month follow-up following the intervention.[39] At baseline, "participants reported poor physical functioning, the majority displayed clinically important psychological distress (66% and 77% for depression and anxiety scales, respectively) and 75% of participants scored above 24 on the catastrophizing scale (p. 647)."[39] At the three-month follow-up, the researchers found an increase in mindfulness practice and a decrease in depression and anxiety scales. Cassidy *et al.* stated, "Improvements in mindfulness over time were associated with improvements in disability and psychological functioning (p. 648)."

MBSR is an effective addition to use in conjunction with CBT because it assists the participants in becoming aware of their negative thoughts and rumination on catastrophic ideas about their pain, anxiety and depressive symptoms.[18] How patients "see" their pain has a significant effect on the severity of their pain.[40] Thus, included within MBSR techniques are virtual body exercises — exercising the synapses, not just the muscles — that also aids in the process of reducing stress and pain.[1,40] Furthermore, mindfulness meditation combined with CBT and guided imagery has been shown to decrease pelvic pain symptoms and increase patients' efforts in self-care techniques.[40]

Any coping skill that aids in the reduction of stress and rumination will aid in the ability to reach deep, restorative sleep.[18,40] CPP causes great difficulty in falling asleep and staying asleep, do not only to the pain but also to the frequent trips to the bathroom if they struggle with PBS or IBS.[20] Research suggests "continuous peripheral noxious stimuli may lead to the development of chronic insomnia (p. 1366)."[41] As discussed earlier, the process of chronic pain and peripheral neuralgias causes changes in the cingulate cortex, which is now being shown to directly relate to the struggle and often inability to sleep.[41] MBSR, hypnosis, guided imagery, and other self-care techniques that aid in calming the whole nervous system will aid in increased and deepened sleep.[40]

References

1. Butler D and Moseley L. *Explain Pain*. Noigroup Publications; 2013.
2. Busch H, Bodin L, Bergström G and Jensen IB. Patterns of sickness absence a decade after pain-related multidisciplinary rehabilitation. *Pain*. 2011;152(8):1727–1733.
3. Sadownik LA, Seal BN and Brotto LA. Provoked vestibulodynia-women's experience of participating in a multidisciplinary vulvodynia program. *J Sex Med*. 2012;9(4):1086–1093.
4. Vlaeyen JWS, Morley S, Linton S, Boersma K and de Jong J. *Pain-Related Fear: Exposure-Based Treatment for Chronic Pain*. Seattle, WA: International Association for the Study of Pain press; 2012.
5. Dawson AP, Schluter PJ, Hodges PW, Stewart S and Turner C. Fear of movement, passive coping, manual handling, and severe or radiating pain increase the likelihood of sick leave due to low back pain. *Pain*. 2011;152(7):1517–1524.
6. Dewitte M, Van Lankveld J and Crombez G. Understanding sexual pain: a cognitive-motivational account. *Pain*. 2011;152(2):251–253.
7. Hidalgo RB and Davidson JR. Posttraumatic stress disorder: epidemiology and health-related considerations. *J Clin Psychiatry*. 2000; 61(Suppl 7):5–13.
8. Keefe FJ and France CR. Pain: Biopsychosocial Mechanisms and Management on JSTOR. 1999. Available on:http://www.jstor.org/stable/20182586?seq=1#page_scan_tab_contents.
9. Wingenfeld K, Hellhammer DH, Schmidt I, Wagner D, Meinlschmidt G and Heim C. HPA axis reactivity in chronic pelvic pain: association with depression. *J Psychosom Obstet Gynaecol*. 2009;30(4): 282–286.
10. Beck JG and Clapp JD. A different kind of co-morbidity: Understanding posttraumatic stress disorder and chronic pain. *Psychol Trauma*. 2011;3(2):101–108.
11. Sharp TJ and Harvey AG. Chronic pain and posttraumatic stress disorder: mutual maintenance? *Clin Psychol Rev*. 2001;21(6):857–877.
12. Organization WH. WHO | The global burden of disease: 2004 update. *WHO* 2008. Available on: http://www.who.int/healthinfo/global_burden_disease/2004_report_update/en/.
13. Gracely RH, Geisser ME, Giesecke T, *et al*. Pain catastrophizing and neural responses to pain among persons with fibromyalgia. *Brain*. 2004;127(Pt 4):835–843.

14. Seminowicz DA and Davis KD. Cortical responses to pain in healthy individuals depends on pain catastrophizing. *Pain.* 2006;120(3): 297–306.

15. Dalpiaz O, Kerschbaumer A, Mitterberger M, Pinggera G, Bartsch G and Strasser H. Chronic pelvic pain in women: still a challenge. *BJU Int.* 2008;102(9):1061–1065.

16. Bair MJ, Robinson RL, Katon W and Kroenke K. Depression and pain comorbidity: a literature review. *Arch Intern Med.* 2003;163(20): 2433–2445.

17. Wegener ST, Castillo RC, Haythornthwaite J, Mackenzie EJ, Bosse MJ and Group LS. Psychological distress mediates the effect of pain on function. *Pain.* 2011;152(6):1349–1357.

18. Segal ZV, Williams JGM and Teasdale JD. *Mindfulness-Based Cognitive Therapy for Depression: A New Approach to Preventing Relapse.* The Guilford Press; 2001.

19. Mattsson M, Wikman M, Dahlgren L and Mattsson B. Physiotherapy as Empowerment — Treating Women with Chronic Pelvic Pain; 2000. Available on: *http://dx.doi.org/10.1080/140381900050175808.*

20. Steege J. *Basic philosophy of the integrated approach in Chronic Pelvic Pain: Evaluation and Management.* Springer; 1997.

21. Thomas K. The mind–body connection: Granny was right, after all, 2011. Available on: http://www.rochester.edu/pr/Review/V59N3/feature2.html.

22. Aydin A, Ahmed K, Zaman I, Khan MS and Dasgupta P. Recurrent urinary tract infections in women. *Int Urogynecol J.* 2015;26(6): 795–804.

23. Jackson JE. Stigma, liminality, and chronic pain: Mind–body borderlands. *American Ethnologist.* 2005;32(3).

24. Bilheimer S and Echenberg RJ. *Secret suffering: how women's sexual and pelvic pain affects their relationships.* Santa Barbara, Calif.: Praeger/ABC-CLIO; 2009.

25. Rusu AC, Pincus T and Morley S. Depressed pain patients differ from other depressed groups: examination of cognitive content in a sentence completion task. *Pain.* 2012;153(9):1898–1904.

26. Payne KA, Binik YM, Pukall CF, Thaler L, Amsel R and Khalifé S. Effects of sexual arousal on genital and non-genital sensation: a comparison of women with vulvar vestibulitis syndrome and healthy controls. *Arch Sex Behav.* 2007;36(2):289–300.

27. Greco CD. Management of adolescent chronic pelvic pain from endometriosis: a pain center perspective. *J Pediatr Adolesc Gynecol.* 2003;16(3 Suppl):S17–S19.
28. Ter Kuile MM and Weijenborg PT. A cognitive-behavioral group program for women with vulvar vestibulitis syndrome (VVS): factors associated with treatment success. *J Sex Marital Ther.* 2006;32(3): 199–213.
29. Price J, Farmer G, Harris J, Hope T, Kennedy S and Mayou R. Attitudes of women with chronic pelvic pain to the gynaecological consultation: a qualitative study. *Bjog.* 2006;113(4):446–452.
30. Moseley L. Unraveling the barriers to reconceptualization of the problem in chronic pain: the actual and perceived ability of patients and health professionals to understand the neurophysiology. *J Pain.* 2003;4(4):184–189.
31. Louw A. Explain Pain. Certification training. National Rehabilitation Hospital, Washington D.C. December 3–4, 2011.
32. Moseley GL. Evidence for a direct relationship between cognitive and physical change during an education intervention in people with chronic low back pain. *Eur J Pain.* 2004;8(1):39–45.
33. Louw A, Puentedura EL and Mintken P. Use of an abbreviated neuroscience education approach in the treatment of chronic low back pain: a case report. *Physiother Theory Pract.* 2012;28(1):50–62.
34. Brotto LA, Bitzer J, Laan E, Leiblum S and Luria M. Women's sexual desire and arousal disorders. *J Sex Med.* 2010;7(1 Pt 2):586–614.
35. Moseley GL and Arntz A. The context of a noxious stimulus affects the pain it evokes. *Pain.* 2007;133(1–3):64–71.
36. Faymonville ME, Laureys S, Degueldre C, *et al.* Neural mechanisms of antinociceptive effects of hypnosis. *Anesthesiology.* 2000;92(5): 1257–1267.
37. Sullivan MJL, Sullivan ME and Adams HM. Stage of chronicity and cognitive correlates of pain-related disability. *Cognitive Behaviour Therapy.* 2002;31(3).
38. Tolle E. *The Power of Now: A Guide to Spiritual Enlightenment.* Namaste Publishing; 2004.
39. Cassidy EL, Atherton RJ, Robertson N, Walsh DA and Gillett R. Mindfulness, functioning and catastrophizing after multidisciplinary pain management for chronic low back pain. *Pain.* 2012;153(3): 644–650.

40. Berna C, Vincent K, Moore J, Tracey I, Goodwin GM and Holmes EA. Presence of mental imagery associated with chronic pelvic pain: a pilot study. *Pain Med.* 2011;12(7):1086–1093.
41. Narita M, Niikura K, Nanjo-Niikura K, *et al.* Sleep disturbances in a neuropathic pain-like condition in the mouse are associated with altered GABAergic transmission in the cingulate cortex. *Pain.* 2011; 152(6):1358–1372.

Chapter 12

Psychodynamic Psychotherapy

Jennifer Schimmel

Psychiatrist and Psychodynamic Therapist, New York, NY 10007

There is evidence that those affected with pelvic pain who are also depressed or anxious may not always respond effectively to standard medical treatment for pelvic pain. In such cases, a multidisciplinary approach to pelvic pain should be considered to treat simultaneously any co-occurring psychological symptoms. Psychodynamic psychotherapy is an abbreviated form of psychoanalysis with fewer patient sessions per week and lasting for a shorter duration. It aims to help patients resolve their emotional difficulties of which they may not be fully aware prior to treatment by employing a variety of techniques to explore patients' feelings. People suffering from pelvic pain often develop psychological symptoms such as anxiety and depression and/or conflicts surrounding sexuality and body image. Psychodynamic psychotherapy has been proven effective in treating this broad range of psychological symptoms and pain syndromes as an adjunct in the treatment of pelvic pain, urological problems, and sexual dysfunction of various causes in both men and women. This chapter will also describe the patient care issues to which a therapist must be sensitive in the psychodynamic evaluation and treatment of patients with pelvic pain.

What is Psychodynamic Psychotherapy?

Psychodynamic psychotherapy is also known as psychoanalytic psychotherapy. The goal of psychodynamic treatment is for the patient to gain an understanding of the basis of his or her feelings, motivations and behavior which are not fully grasped by the patient before the treatment.[1]

One should note that, while many scoff at the mere mention of psychoanalysis and Sigmund Freud, one of its founders, many varied schools of thought have developed from observations of the differences between theory and technique. These different strains have shaped the practice of modern day psychoanalysis and psychodynamic psychotherapy. Both treatments have been disparaged by obsolete and inaccurate portrayals in the media, popular culture, and, not least of all, outdated psychology textbooks. The clichés are all too familiar: the psychoanalyst as austere and silent clinician, only interested in the exploration of sex and aggression; the psychoanalyst as bored, distracted, or sleepy while his patient — shown lying on a couch — drones on about his or her experiences. Despite being a staple of television drama and *New Yorker* magazine cartoons, this portrayal is simply untrue.[1]

Psychodynamic psychotherapy is an abbreviated form of psychoanalysis. Psychodynamic psychotherapy patients meet with the therapist once or twice per week instead of three to five times, and the timespan of treatment is generally shorter than that of psychoanalysis.[1] Psychodynamic psychotherapy can be either an open ended treatment with no predetermined number of sessions or can be time limited.[2]

Psychodynamic therapy is distinguished from many other psychotherapies by the idea of an "unconscious" part of the mind. Essentially, the unconscious means the part of one's mind containing those thoughts, feelings, wishes and fantasies that are not readily accessible just by actively shifting one's attention or focus to them. They are essentially out of one's awareness. In contrast, the "conscious" part of the mind contains the elements that are readily accessible to us just by shifting our attention to them. Often, conscious aspects of one's experience become unconscious because they make one feel uncomfortable or vulnerable in some way. "They make us want to look away."[1] Unfortunately, looking away is problematic. When one attempts to avert one's gaze from unpleasant thoughts and feelings, those thoughts and feelings persist and survive. One only loses touch with what one really knows and deeply feels about oneself and the important people in one's life.

Distinctive Features of Psychodynamic Technique

Blagys and Hilsenroth conducted a literature review of the *PsychLit* database of all studies that compared the process and technique of psychodynamic psychotherapy with that of cognitive-behavioral therapy (CBT).[3] They identified seven areas — which Shedler subsequently described — that reliably distinguish psychodynamic psychotherapy from CBT. They also believe these seven areas correlate with what makes psychodynamic psychotherapy effective.

1. *Focus on feeling and the expression of emotion*: Psychodynamic psychotherapists try to help patients understand and express their hidden feelings. It is not enough to understand oneself from an intellectual perspective. Many people know, from an intellectual perspective, the reasons for their difficulties, yet this understanding does not help them change. It is the integration of intellectual and emotional experiencing that deeply heals problems and improves symptoms.[1]
2. *Exploration of attempts to avoid distressing thoughts and feelings*: Emotions are often painful; therefore, there is a natural and frequently unintentional inclination to try to avoid them, whether in a therapy session or in real life. In therapy, such avoidance can take the form of a patient's changing the subject to something less painful during a session or even a patient's arriving late to sessions to avoid talking about things.

(Unlike many other branches of medicine, psychodynamic psychotherapy appointments must start promptly and end promptly to encourage patients to confront such efforts to avoid the unpleasant thoughts and feelings.) The psychodynamic therapist notices and points these things out to patients to help patients to realize what they might be avoiding and how they do so without intentionally meaning to do so.

3. *Identification of recurring themes and patterns*: An example of this may be someone who repeatedly sabotages himself or herself, perhaps due to suppressed feelings of guilt, when he or she is close to achieving a particular success. A psychodynamic therapist would help the patient to recognize this pattern of behavior in himself or herself and help him or her delve into the feelings that underlie the pattern of behavior so that this pattern is no longer necessary.

4. *Discussion of past experience (i.e. developmental focus)*: It is a tenet of psychodynamic theory that people are shaped by their childhood/adolescent experiences and, further, that people unknowingly re-create or repeat in the present those past experiences that are tied to their hidden and unresolved feelings. By understanding one's past and how it affects one's present feelings, relationships, and behavior, one can free oneself from the bonds of the past and "live more fully in the present."[1]

5. *Focus on Interpersonal relations*: There is a strong focus on the patient's interpersonal relationships and how they affect the patient's personality and self-concept.

6. *Focus on the therapy relationship*: Just as there are recurring themes in a person's life, one's relationship patterns tend to recur within the therapy itself with the therapist. A patient who tends to distrust people in his or her life will often grow distrustful of the therapist. A patient who has difficulty with authority figures, who perhaps has difficulty staying employed, can come to see the therapist as an authority figure and experience him or her in a negative and controlling way. The therapy becomes a "relationship laboratory" of sorts where the

therapist and patient can observe and work through the patient's relationship patterns. This technique is central to psychodynamic psychotherapy and it can create significant and lasting change in a patient.

7. *Exploration of wishes and fantasies*: As noted above, exploring otherwise unconscious feelings, desires and fears can help patients better understand themselves. These can be accessed through a process called free association, where patients allow their thoughts to roam freely from topic to topic during sessions. The connections between the topics can be as revealing as the thoughts themselves. This process will be discussed below. These aspects of one's feelings can also be explored by examining the thoughts one ascribes to the content of one's daydreams and dreams.[1]

Differences between Psychodynamic Psychotherapy and CBT

In addition to discussing the distinctive features of psychodynamic technique, one can better understand psychodynamic psychotherapy by contrasting psychodynamic psychotherapy and CBT. They are both psychological therapies that may be used, in varied situations, as adjunctive treatments to pelvic pain, but psychodynamic psychotherapy and CBT "manage feelings" differently. In the practice of psychodynamic psychotherapy, patients are encouraged to unearth their feelings, and significant time is devoted to deepening and understanding feelings in order to gain mastery over one's "wishes, desires, fears, and anxieties." CBT attempts to "control, manage, reduce, moderate or explain feeling in order to decrease stress and convey a more reality based sense of self."[3] Blagys and Hilsenroth maintain that CBT centers on relieving a focused set of a patient's symptoms to reduce stress while psychodynamic psychotherapy emphasizes the growth of those psychological capabilities which affect a patient's view of oneself and of others, thereby effecting symptom relief. For Shedler, a successful treatment not only reduces symptoms such as depression and anxiety but also adds something.[1] That something may be the ability to have more fulfilling friendships or to make better use of one's particular talents or to have more satisfying sexual relationships, etc.

Why Psychodynamic Psychotherapy?

Why should we expect a psychotherapeutic approach such as psychodynamic psychotherapy to be a helpful adjunct in the treatment of pelvic pain? One reason is that there are conditions suited to treatment with psychodynamic psychotherapy that co-occur in the context of pelvic pain. Depression and anxiety are extremely common in people who have pelvic pain as well as people who have chronic pain in other locations, further negatively affecting their quality of life.[4–8] Suffering from depression and anxiety in the context of chronic pelvic pain (CPP) can lead to interpersonal difficulties, from marital problems to professional problems.[5]

The sources and causes of depression and anxiety in pelvic pain are likely multifold. There are neurobiological reasons stemming from certain commonalities of pain, depression, and anxiety. Common areas in the brain are triggered. The same part of the brain is activated when someone is depressed and anxious as when someone is in pain. Similarly, the neurotransmitters norepinephrine and serotonin also mediate all three of these states.[9]

Being anxious or depressed can intensify one's perception of pain and make one's pain more difficult to tolerate.[10,11] There are orthopedic reasons that connect anxiety and pelvic pain. The pelvic floor comprises many different muscles, the nerves which control these muscles, and the connective tissue and ligaments which join these muscles. Muscle difficulties (including contraction of different muscle groups) and irritation of critically located nerves are associated with different pain symptoms in both men and women.[12] Stress and anxiety can increase muscle tension in all parts of the body, including in the pelvic floor. This can result in pelvic pain.

There is significant medical evidence for the connection between mind and body in the context of pelvic pain.

Dellon *et al.* conducted a study to evaluate the effectiveness of regional pudendal nerve resection — a surgical procedure — for patients with pelvic pain.[13] They expected to find that pudendal nerve resection could help those patients where non-surgical attempts at pain management such as myofascial trigger point release and medication management of pelvic pain had failed. Astoundingly, they found that the biggest predictor of failure for this surgical procedure was a patient's untreated depression and anxiety. In other words, for those patients who were found to be anxious and depressed, cutting a nerve associated with the transmission of signals of pelvic pain to the brain did not improve pelvic pain. They began recommending that evaluation and treatment of psychological symptoms occur pre-operatively.[13]

Psychological reasons play a role as well in pelvic pain. An arduous search for pain relief can be associated with feelings of hopelessness, helplessness, and depression.[14] People naturally tend to attribute meaning to their pain.[15] Sometimes it can be hard to know for certain when the pain will end and how the pain will affect one's life. People also wonder what their pain means about them. Patients may question themselves. "What is wrong with me?" "Will the pain get worse?" "How am I ever going to get better?" "Who will ever love me like this"?[15] Pelvic pain can also affect one's feelings about his or her body. For example, women with vestibulodynia have a more negative body image during sexual activity when there is associated decreased sexual satisfaction, decreased sexual function and pain during intercourse. Women with pain during intercourse have more negative feelings and resentment toward their own genitals.[16]

Although there are many people with pelvic pain who do not have a history of emotional, physical or sexual trauma, there is a higher-than-average association of chronic pain including pelvic pain with abuse.[17] For this reason, it is an important factor to consider in treating people with pelvic pain. McCauley *et al.* assessed 1,931 women of various ages, marital, educational, and socioeconomic backgrounds in four community-based, internal medicine practices. Twenty-two percent of these patients reported a history of childhood physical or sexual abuse, and these women had higher scores for depression, anxiety and low self-esteem. Further, 23.5% of the women with a history of abuse reported pelvic pain, but only 11.2% of the women without a history of abuse did so.

Given that multiple studies have found that patients with pelvic pain have high rates of depression and anxiety and that some patients also have a history of sexual and non-sexual abuse disproportionately associated with psychiatric comorbidities, a multidisciplinary approach to pelvic pain is warranted. Pelvic pain patients should also be screened for psychiatric symptoms and treated for these symptoms, in addition to the evaluation and management of their physical symptoms. Not addressing such psychological problems can hinder the treatment of pelvic pain.[11] Depression, anxiety, low self-esteem, effects of sexual trauma, negative body image and the negative meanings people ascribe to their pain are all psychological aspects that can be better understood and worked through using psychodynamic psychotherapy.

For reasons similar to those noted above, psychodynamic psychotherapy can also be a helpful adjunct in the treatment of several urological disorders in both men and women. Patients with disorders including chronic urinary tract infections (UTIs), overactive bladder (OAB), stress and urge incontinence, and interstitial cystitis (IC) typically experience symptoms such as urinary frequency and urgency; increased nighttime urination; pain in the urethra, bladder, or pelvis; and urinary incontinence.[12] These symptoms can result from chronic inflammation, muscle tightness or muscle weakness, which in turn are often exacerbated by psychological conditions like depression, anxiety and chronic stress.[12] A study by Ito *et al.* sought to determine whether major depression was a risk factor for bladder, bowel, and sexual dysfunction.[18] They found that in both men and women with depression, the rate of urinary urgency and urinary incontinence was increased.

A literature review by Sakakibara *et al.* was undertaken to evaluate the effect of depression and anxiety on bladder function.[19] They found OAB symptoms were more common in patients with depression and in patients with anxiety. The most significant finding was that these patients experienced increased bladder sensation which was the most common cause of their problems. They believe that this increased bladder sensation relates to biological changes in areas of the brain with overlapping functions; these areas are under the control of similar neurotransmitters which regulate both emotions and functions pertaining to urination. They conclude that "bladder dysfunction in depression and anxiety presumably reflects that the bladder is under emotional control" and that "depression and anxiety are risk factors for bladder dysfunction."[19] Psychodynamic psychotherapy has been shown to be highly effective in the treatment of depression and anxiety. These psychological conditions often relate to urological symptoms. Thus, it is likely that psychodynamic psychotherapy could be a helpful adjunct in the treatment of urological symptoms.

It is well understood that sexual dysfunction is often exacerbated by psychological issues. Psychodynamic psychotherapy can be a helpful adjunct in the treatment of sexual dysfunction including disorders of libido and orgasm in men and women and male difficulty in achieving and maintaining an erection. Sexual dysfunction in both men and women can relate to a variety of psychological issues such as coexisting depression or anxiety. Psychodynamic psychotherapy can help to alleviate symptoms of depression and anxiety and therefore increase sexual functioning.[1]

In addition, this type of therapy is extremely valuable in helping patients understand and work through their inhibitions and negative beliefs, whether conscious or unconscious, about their sexuality. For example, despite consciously wanting to improve their sexual functioning, some patients may unconsciously believe that they should not enjoy sex. Sexual dysfunction can present in the context about guilt over having an extramarital affair.[2] People are also raised with a variety of beliefs about sexuality, which may become unconscious and thus not easily accessible to a patient at the onset of psychodynamic treatment. It is only after treatment has unearthed these beliefs that patients may realize that they have a lot of shame and guilt about being sexually active, which shame and guilt may worsen sexual dysfunction.

When someone develops sexual dysfunction in the context of an established relationship, it is important to understand the changes in that relationship. Has the patient developed resentment toward the partner which could be contributing to sexual dysfunction? Unresolved feelings from childhood may result in a lack of interest in sex or difficulty achieving an orgasm in women, or lack of interest in sex, difficulty achieving or maintaining an erection or difficulty with orgasm in men.[2]

In "An Update of the International Society of Sexual Medicine's Guidelines for the Diagnosis and Treatment of Premature Ejaculation (PE)", Althof *et al.* noted many psychological and interpersonal factors which could contribute to PE.[20] Some of these included: ideas internalized about sex from childhood; depression; performance anxiety; body image; and a history of sexual abuse. In addition, relationship problems such as difficulty with intimacy and conflict with a partner could play a role. They also note that the development of PE could then exacerbate the initial psychological difficulties.

The majority of men and women with sexual dysfunction do not have a history of childhood physical or sexual abuse. However, for those patients with a history of childhood trauma there is a higher prevalence of sexual dysfunction than in the general population.[20] A study by Tekin *et al.* aimed to evaluate the effect of childhood physical and sexual trauma on sexual functioning in patients with social anxiety disorder and coexisting depression.[21] They found that depressed men and women with social anxiety disorder who have a history of either childhood physical or sexual traumatic experiences were at greater risk for sexual dysfunction.

How Effective is Psychodynamic Psychotherapy?

Psychodynamic psychotherapy is very effective in treating a wide range of psychological symptoms including depression and anxiety.

Psychodynamic psychotherapy has also been shown to be helpful in treating pain syndromes including pelvic pain. As noted above, physical and sexual abuse is more common in people with pelvic pain. As a result of this abuse, people can develop detrimental personality characteristics such as intermittent depression, anxiety, difficulty with emotional regulation, low self-esteem, poor body image, and interpersonal difficulties.[22] Psychodynamic psychotherapy has shown dramatic efficacy in treating personality issues.[1]

Several research articles depict the effectiveness of psychodynamic psychotherapy. Shedler published one such article, reporting on multiple meta-analytic studies aimed at determining the effectiveness of psychodynamic psychotherapy on a variety of psychiatric symptoms and diagnoses. (A "meta-analysis" is designed to make the results of different studies comparable by converting findings into a "common metric, allowing findings to be aggregated or pooled across studies".[1])

The results are impressive. One meta-analysis included 23 randomized controlled trials, a total of 1,431 patients. Patients had a broad range of psychiatric symptoms and diagnoses. Symptoms were measured at the end of the treatment and then nine months or greater after the patients ended psychodynamic psychotherapy. The effect size for general symptom improvement was very high, at 0.97. (In these trials, "effect size" measures the improvement of patients' symptoms who received psychodynamic psychotherapy compared to a control group receiving no treatment or a different kind of treatment. The larger the effect size, the more effective psychodynamic psychotherapy is in treating various symptoms. With respect to the scale, an "effect size" of 0.5 means that the treatment under evaluation is moderately effective; 0.2 means a low effectiveness and 1.0 means a very high effect.[1])

Continuing with the trials noted immediately above, at nine months post-treatment the effect size for general symptom improvement increased to 1.51. Effect sizes were examined by condition. Psychodynamic psychotherapy had an effect size of

1.08 with respect to anxiety symptoms, which increased to 1.35 at follow-up. For depressive symptoms, it was 0.59, increasing to 0.98 at follow-up. For somatic symptoms, i.e. different pain symptoms, the effect size was 0.81 at the end of the study and it increased to 2.21 post-treatment, an amazingly large improvement. (Improvement was also seen in symptoms associated with personality disorders.) This observed increase in post-treatment efficacy is a unique finding to psychodynamic psychotherapy and is not found in other psychotherapeutic treatment modalities. This continuing improvement or "sleeper effect" has been replicated many times in different studies of psychodynamic psychotherapy. Shedler proposes that "psychodynamic psychotherapy sets in motion psychological processes that lead to ongoing change, even after therapy has ended."[1]

Another paper, authored by Abbass *et al.*, looked at 21 studies of psychodynamic psychotherapy.[23] They found similar findings to Shedler *et al.* as described above. Of note, one of the studies was a randomized control trial of psychodynamic psychotherapy for urethral syndrome and pelvic pain. Patients were randomly assigned either to receive psychodynamic psychotherapy plus the standard medical treatment or to receive standard medical treatment alone. Patients assigned to the psychodynamic psychotherapy plus medical treatment group had a decrease in urinary symptoms and pelvic pain. Seventy percent of patients in the psychodynamic psychotherapy group were in remission four years later. In this same study, symptoms such as anxiety, depression and hostility showed improvement in the psychodynamic psychotherapy group at the end of treatment. At the four-year-follow-up, depression and hostility measures were still improved.[23,24]

There are many other studies which show improvement in psychological symptoms including depression, anxiety, interpersonal problems, and pain syndromes.[25] Abbass *et al.* found psychodynamic psychotherapy to be efficacious in the treatment of somatic symptoms including dermatological, neurological, cardiovascular, respiratory, gastrointestinal, musculoskeletal, genitourinary (GU) and immunological systems.[23] Psychodynamic psychotherapy also improved social–occupational functioning, treatment compliance and led to a decrease in healthcare utilization.

Psychodynamic Evaluation for Pelvic Pain

Although the treatment and evaluation section as written below focuses primarily on pelvic pain, these principles can also be applied when evaluating and treating patients with urinary problems and sexual dysfunction. A patient with pelvic pain may come with mixed feelings to his or her initial meeting with a therapist. He or she may worry that they are being referred to a psychotherapist because his or her doctor or physical therapist thinks that the patient's pain is not "real" (and therefore not treatable). Patients with this concern feel resentful and uncomfortable about seeing a mental health professional. A psychotherapist must confront and dispel this myth during the evaluation itself, because otherwise a successful evaluation and treatment is unlikely. It is important to reassure the patient that there are real factors behind their pain, whether it is a problem with the pelvic floor muscles, nerve problems or inflammation in or around the pelvic organs that are causing the patient pain.[26]

One must understand the characteristics of the patient's pelvic pain. What makes the pain better or worse? What treatments have been tried and the helpfulness of these treatments? The therapist should ask about psychological symptoms such as depression and anxiety.[26] The therapist should also ask about other health problems.

As discussed previously, symptoms such as anxiety or depression can result from being in pain and can also relate to what being in pain means to a patient. It is sometimes helpful to explain the pain, anxiety and tension cycle; the anxiety or stress a patient feels can increase muscle tension and aggravate pain. Stressful thoughts and feelings can worsen anxiety which can worsen pain.[15] Once something is known about the pelvic pain characteristics and psychiatric symptoms the evaluation can broaden.

A psychodynamic evaluation differs from a typical medical intake and initial interview in that it is often more free form, without a checklist of symptoms. The details about a patient's pelvic pain and psychiatric symptoms may come out only at the end of the evaluation. Patients sometimes start talking about their other struggles first. It can be helpful to follow the patient's lead as to what the patient chooses to be more important to tell a therapist first. When the patient defers a discussion about pelvic pain or psychiatric symptoms, the therapist should first develop a better sense of the patient and his or her struggles before proceeding on to other parts of the evaluation. Why is the patient seeking a psychotherapy evaluation now? Did their doctor or physical therapist recommend it? Does the patient also feel it is important? Has something recently changed in the patient's life that has prompted them to seek a psychotherapy evaluation at this particular time? What does the patient desire from psychodynamic treatment? Does the patient want symptom relief from depression or anxiety? Does the patient want to know himself or herself more deeply; master a specific difficulty; or achieve a specific life goal?

In his chapter on "Treating the Patient with Pelvic Pain," Dr. Mark Elliott notes the importance of understanding a patient's personality style, psychosocial factors, and stressors. Additional areas of understanding should involve relationship issues including sexual problems. In a sensitive way, the psychotherapist should also ask about any history of emotional, physical or sexual abuse, especially because of the observed role of such abuse in some patients' pelvic pain.[26]

It is also important to obtain information about educational level, employment history and current living situation. How do symptoms related to either pain or emotional issues interfere with a patient's ability to work and form emotionally intimate, fulfilling relationships? Finally, an understanding of past psychiatric treatments is important. What types of therapy has the patient undergone and for how long? What was a person's relationship with the therapist like? What results were accomplished? When and why did the treatment end? Has the patient ever been on any psychiatric medications?[22]

Psychodynamic Treatment as an Adjunct to the Treatment of Pelvic Pain

There is much history to be collected from patients, and it can be hard to distinguish the end of the evaluation and the start of treatment. Empathy and curiosity on the therapist's part go a long way in making the patient feel comfortable and able to open up and share his or her feelings and history. A psychodynamic psychotherapy consultation may take multiple sessions. Sometimes, some of the information mentioned in the above evaluation section, depending on the patient, cannot be gathered until a treatment is underway as some patients are not aware of how they deeply feel and what is truly bothering them.

As noted above in the discussion of psychodynamic technique, the order in which patients recall and relate memories, feelings and thoughts can give the psychotherapist a good sense of what the patient is struggling with consciously and unconsciously. The order in which things come to mind may seem random but it is actually quite meaningful. Things that are recalled in close proximity to each other are often related in an unconscious way.[2] For example, a patient could be talking about her fears about beginning psychotherapy and then immediately afterwards talk about the sadness she feels about her friend moving away to a new city. Perhaps, one of the anxieties this patient feels about being in psychotherapy is a fear about loss, as described by the sadness of a friend moving away. Open-ended story telling is important both in the psychodynamic evaluation and as a technique in the treatment phase. While the seven features of psychodynamic psychotherapy described above are the cornerstone of psychodynamic treatment, one must note that psychodynamic treatment is highly individualized to the difficulties of each patient. Below are some illustrations of how some of the difficulties with which patients with pelvic pain may struggle can be understood and treated with psychodynamic psychotherapy techniques and concepts.

Pelvic pain is often caused by a medical problem such as nerve pain and/or muscle tension as previously discussed, but anxiety or depression can exacerbate the pain.[12,15] In that case, to lessen the pain psychodynamically, one must understand the psychological causes of a patient's anxiety. For example, by delving into the events of the patient's life when the pelvic pain began or became exacerbated, a therapist can learn whether the pain developed or was worsened in the context of a significant life event about which the patient, even unknowingly, feels some conflict, i.e. ambivalent feelings.

Feelings are complicated, perhaps more complicated than people would like to admit. In his 2006 article, Shedler talks about how people often have complex and even contradictory feelings about the people and events in their lives.[27] People often feel badly about this because they expect themselves to feel only one way. For example, people feel guilty about having both loving and aggressive feelings toward loved ones. In order to rid themselves of the seemingly distasteful or guilt-inducing feelings, people look away from these feelings, which get tucked away in the unconscious but expressed elsewhere, even in the mind–body connection. Hypothetically, a patient's pelvic pain could worsen in the context of getting married if they feel ambivalent or have mixed feelings about getting married and cannot access or express the complexity of these feelings.

Emotional intimacy is another area often marked by complex feelings. A patient who has conflictual, or ambivalent, feelings about intimacy may desire an intimate relationship but yet do things to sabotage intimacy. Such a patient may continually choose partners who are emotionally unavailable as a way to avoid intimacy.[27] Perhaps, a person's pelvic pain is observed to worsen in the context of him or her developing a closer relationship with someone more emotionally present and available. Although it might feel good initially to such a person to be in a healthier relationship, the expectation of deeper intimacy could also create anxiety. An increase in anxiety might cause the person to tense up his or her pelvic floor muscles thus creating or making pelvic pain worse. Psychodynamic psychotherapy can help such a patient understand and tolerate these complicated feelings.

By helping a patient work through his or her conflict related to difficulty with intimacy, the patient can have healthier interpersonal relationships which create less anxiety. If anxiety lessens, the pelvic pain can lessen.[15]

There are also some people who have what Wise and Anderson call "pleasure anxiety". They describe people with pelvic pain who associate the feeling of pleasure or safety with something bad happening. This fear can develop when one unexpectedly experiences something traumatic — such as the death of a loved one — when one is feeling otherwise happy and secure.

Afterwards, something good happening in one's life would evoke anxiety and tension in the pelvic floor, thus creating or exacerbating pelvic pain. These authors also note that when the feeling of pleasure or safety is too anxiety provoking, holding on to pelvic pain can serve the function of warding off pleasure. However, such suffering of physical pain is an unhealthy adaptation to one's anxiety; psychodynamic psychotherapy is well suited to help a patient examine and unravel such unconscious problems.

People are raised with different ideas about sexuality. Some people feel guilt and shame about their sexuality. They can develop intense anxiety about being sexually active. Such feelings can exacerbate pelvic pain and can also lead to diminished sexual pleasure and sexual functioning.[15] There are many people who have conflictual feelings about sexuality who have never been abused. However, there is a higher rate of history of sexual abuse in people who have pelvic pain as compared to the history of people without pelvic pain.[17] In his description of psychodynamic psychotherapy in people with pelvic pain, Dr. Elliott notes that people with a history of sexual abuse often do not respond well to other forms of psychotherapy such as CBT. In addition, some of these people do not have a good response to the standard medical treatment of pelvic pain. He notes that some people who have been abused are unconsciously fearful of getting better. Perhaps, they believe that without pelvic pain they may feel obligated to engage sexually with a partner and that expectation may be very frightening. He notes that psychodynamic psychotherapy can help people work through their feelings about their sexual trauma, which can allow medical treatments to be more helpful such that pelvic pain can then subside.

It cannot be repeated too often that just because there is a strong interplay and feedback loop between physical pain and emotional issues it does not mean that the emotional issues make the physical pain any less "real." Dellon *et al.* discussion above — on the role of untreated anxiety and depression on the failure of surgical pelvic pain management — well demonstrates the arbitrariness in trying to separate and distinguish what the human brain perceives from what the human mind thinks and feels.[13]

In their journal article about the experiences of women undergoing physical therapy for a variety of orthopedic problems, Schacter, Stalker and Teram describe some of the difficulties these women experience undergoing physical therapy. They interviewed 27 survivors of childhood sexual abuse. Information about their experience in physical therapy and suggestions they had that could improve their experience was gathered. Many of these women described having difficulties being touched even in areas such as their feet. The authors note that many of these women experienced "intense feelings such as fear, anxiety, terror, grief, or anger, that suddenly and without warning surfaced after being triggered by some aspect of physical therapy."[28]

Consider myofascial trigger point release, a non-surgical treatment for pelvic pain, performed by a physical therapist. This treatment may involve accessing the pelvic floor muscles through the vagina or anus.[12] One might imagine that this could be quite traumatic for someone with a history of sexual abuse. One could reasonably infer from the Schacter study that undergoing myofascial trigger point release physical therapy might create similar or even more extreme reactions in patients. Perhaps, some of these patients would not be able to fully participate in this essential treatment until some of these issues of abuse had been worked through in a psychodynamic psychotherapy.

Conclusions

This chapter has been a simplified explanation of psychodynamic psychotherapy, including its theoretical underpinnings and its basic techniques, and how it differs from other psychotherapeutic modalities such as CBT. Common psychological symptoms which can occur in both women and men who may suffer from a range of anatomical problems that can result in pelvic pain, urinary problems and sexual dysfunction were discussed. Examples of such symptoms are depression; anxiety; and emotional conflicts such as guilt, shame, interpersonal difficulties and low self-esteem. It is hard to refute that, while pain may have a clear anatomic etiology, there is clear evidence for a mind–body connection. There is substantial confirmation in the literature, as discussed in this chapter, that surgical and non-surgical treatment of pelvic pain is less effective for treating pain when these psychological issues have not been addressed. Psychodynamic psychotherapy can be highly effective in treating people with such difficulties as evidenced in the literature. The psychodynamic evaluation and management of patients with pelvic pain has also been outlined.

People seeking psychodynamic psychotherapy should expect more than just alleviation of psychological symptoms such as anxiety and depression. With completed treatment, they should expect to gain "something more". The "something more" might be: the ability to experience more pleasure and satisfaction from interpersonal relationships; an improved, reality-based self-esteem and greater satisfaction from one's accomplishments; an enhanced creativity; or greater enjoyment of one's sexuality, etc. While the durations of psychodynamic psychotherapies vary, some people may argue that it is too time consuming or expensive. However, such arguments against the cost effectiveness of psychodynamic psychotherapy ignore the evidence showing that patients change on a deep level such that even after termination of psychodynamic psychotherapy, patients continue to improve emotionally to the extent that they may not need to return to a therapist for refresher courses or work on other issues.

This chapter was written with the hope that women and men who suffer from pelvic pain and dysfunction — whether urinary or gynecological in origin — and their medical treatment providers might recognize the need for and value of a multidisciplinary approach to pelvic pain, urinary problems or sexual dysfunction that incorporates the treatment of patients' psychological issues. Referring patients to mental health providers trained in psychodynamic psychotherapy can be a helpful adjunctive measure in their treatment regimen.

References

1. Shedler J. The efficacy of psychodynamic psychotherapy. *Am Psychol.* 2010;65(2):98–109.
2. Gabbard GO. *Psychodynamic Psychiatry in Clinical Practice.* Amer Psychiatric Pub; 2014.
3. Blagys M and Hilsenroth M. Distinctive Features of Short-? Term psychodynamic interpersonal psychotherapy: a review of the comparative psychotherapy process literature. *Clin Psychol Sci Pract.* 2000;7(2):167–188.
4. de Heer EW, Gerrits MM, Beekman AT, *et al.* The association of depression and anxiety with pain: a study from NESDA. *PLoS One.* 2014;9(10):e106907.
5. Romao AP, Gorayeb R, Romao GS, *et al.* High levels of anxiety and depression have a negative effect on quality of life of women with chronic pelvic pain. *Int J Clin Pract.* 2009;63(5):707–711.
6. Walker E, Katon W, Harrop-Griffiths J, Holm L, Russo J and Hickok LR. Relationship of chronic pelvic pain to psychiatric diagnoses and childhood sexual abuse. *Am J Psychiatry.* 1988;145(1):75–80.
7. Walker EA, Katon WJ, Hansom J, *et al.* Psychiatric diagnoses and sexual victimization in women with chronic pelvic pain. *Psychosomatics.* 1995;36(6):531–540.
8. Fry RP, Crisp AH, Beard RW and McGuigan S. Psychosocial aspects of chronic pelvic pain, with special reference to sexual abuse. A study of 164 women. *Postgrad Med J.* 1993;69(813):566–574.
9. Bair MJ, Robinson RL, Eckert GJ, Stang PE, Croghan TW and Kroenke K. Impact of pain on depression treatment response in primary care. *Psychosom Med.* 2004;66(1):17–22.

10. Holzberg AD, Robinson ME, Geisser ME and Gremillion HA. The effects of depression and chronic pain on psychosocial and physical functioning. *Clin J Pain*. 1996;12(2):118–125.
11. Meltzer-Brody S and Leserman J. Psychiatric comorbidity in women with chronic pelvic pain. *CNS Spectr*. 2011;16(2):29–35.
12. Stein A. *Heal Pelvic Pain: The Proven Stretching, Strengthening, and Nutrition Program for Relieving Pain, Incontinence, & I.B.S, and Other Symptoms Without Surgery*. McGraw-Hill Education; 2008.
13. Dellon AL, Coady D and Harris D. Pelvic pain of pudendal nerve origin: surgical outcomes and learning curve lessons. *J Reconstr Microsurg*. 2015;31(4):283–290.
14. Turk DC, Audette J, Levy RM, Mackey SC and Stanos S. Assessment and treatment of psychosocial comorbidities in patients with neuropathic pain. *Mayo Clin Proc*. 2010;85(3 Suppl):S42–S50.
15. Wise D and Anderson R. A Headache In the Pelvis. 2003; Available on: http://www.prostatitis.org/aheadacheinthepelvis.html.
16. Maille DL, Bergeron S and Lambert B. Body image in women with primary and secondary provoked vestibulodynia: a controlled study. *J Sex Med*. 2015;12(2):505–515.
17. McCauley J, Kern DE, Kolodner K, *et al*. Clinical characteristics of women with a history of childhood abuse: unhealed wounds. *JAMA*. 1997;277(17):1362–1368.
18. Ito T, Sakakibara R, Shimizu E, *et al*. Is Major Depression a Risk for Bladder, Bowel, and Sexual Dysfunction? *LUTS: Lower Urinary Tract Symptoms*. 2012;4(2):87–95.
19. Sakakibara R, Ito T, Yamamoto T, *et al*. Depression, Anxiety and the Bladder. *LUTS: Lower Urinary Tract Symptoms*. 2013;5(3):109–120.
20. Althof SE, McMahon CG, Waldinger MD, *et al*. an update of the international society of sexual medicine's guidelines for the diagnosis and treatment of premature ejaculation (PE). *Sex Med*. 2014;2(2):60–90.
21. Tekin A, Meric C, Sagbilge E, *et al*. The relationship between childhood sexual/physical abuse and sexual dysfunction in patients with social anxiety disorder. *Nord J Psychiatry*. 2016;70(2):88–92.
22. Association AP. Practice Guideline for the Psychiatric Evaluation of Adults. 2006; 2nd. Available on: http://psychiatryonline.org/pb/assets/raw/sitewide/practice_guidelines/guidelines/psychevaladults.pdf.

23. Abbass A, Town J and Driessen E. Intensive short-term dynamic psychotherapy: a systematic review and meta-analysis of outcome research. *Harv Rev Psychiatry*. 2012;20(2):97–108.

24. Baldoni F, Baldaro B and Trombini G. Psychotherapeutic Perspectives in Urethral Syndrome. *Stress Medicine*. 1995;11(1).

25. Gerber AJ, Kocsis JH, Milrod BL, *et al.* A quality-based review of randomized controlled trials of psychodynamic psychotherapy. *Am J Psychiatry*. 2011;168(1):19–28.

26. Elliott M. *Treating the Patient with Pelvic Pain in Psychological Approaches to Pain Management, Second Edition: A Practitioner's Handbook*. The Guilford Press; 2002.

27. Shedler J. That was then, this is now: An introduction to contemporary pscyhodynamic therapy. 2006; 2011. Available on:http://www.jonathanshedler.com/PDFs/Shedler%20(2006)%20That%20was%20then,%20this%20is%20now%20R9.pdf.

28. Schachter CL, Stalker CA and Teram E. Toward sensitive practice: issues for physical therapists working with survivors of childhood sexual abuse. *Phys Ther*. 1999;79(3):248–261; discussion 262–249.

Index

A

abdominis, 8
abdominal/intestinal massage, 156
Achillea fillipendulina (fernleaf
  yarrow), 38
alanine, 61
alkaline urine, 22
Allium sativum (garlic), 32
aloe vera (aloe), 38
Althaea officinalis (marshmallow),
  24
amenorrhea, 12
Ammi visnaga (khella), 36
Angelica sinensis, 64
anxiety, 186
Apium graveolens (celery), 36
Arctostaphylos uva ursi
  (Bearberry), 48
arginine, 34
asana, 190, 194
Ashwagandha (*Withania
  sominifera*), 70

B

Bandhas, 189
benign prostatic hyperplasia
  (BPH), 14, 28, 60, 118
biofeedback, 168, 173, 177
bowel and GI disturbances, 76
Bryophyllum pinnatum (air
  plant), 25
buchu, 22

C

calcium, 73
celiac disease, 92
Centaurium erythraea (common
  centaury), 38
Centella asiatica (Gotu Kola), 34,
  57
chronic orchialgia, 118
chronic pelvic pain (CPP), 135,
  186, 223, 231
chronic prostatitis and chronic
  Pelvic Pain, 117

Cinnamomum spp (cinnamon), 26
clitoradynia, 12
connective tissue mobilization, 149
constipation, 9, 11, 17, 176
cornsilk, 28
Cornus, 57
couch grass, 28
cranberry (*Vaccinium macrocarpon*), 47
cryotherapy, 166
cup therapy, 154
curculigo, 57
cystine stones, 75
cystocele, 134

D
depression, 249
detrusor overactivity, 175
DHEA, 63, 68–69
diindolemethane (DIM), 53
Dirgha, 188
D-Mannose, 47
dry needling (DN) therapy, 155
dysfunctional voiding, 175
dysmenorrhea, 12, 103, 186

E
Echinacea angustifolia (purple coneflower), 23
Elymus repens (couch grass), 24
endometriosis, 103
Ephedra sinica (ma huang), 26
epididymitis, 118
epimedium and icariin, 67
Equisetum spp (horsetail), 36
erectile disorder or ejaculation problems, 13

erectile dysfunction (ED), 14, 32, 122, 137, 179
Eryngium yuccifolium (rattlesnake master), 24

F
female orgasm disorder, 64
female pelvic pain, 56, 121
female sexual dysfunction, 62, 120
fibroids, 103
fibromyalgia, 186
Four Examinations, 8

G
Ganoderma lucidum (GL), 51
gardenia, 57
garlic (*Allium sativum*), 46
GI dysfunction, 10
Gingko biloba, 63
Ginkgo biloba leaf extract, 34
glutamic acid, 61
glycine, 61

H
H. Canadensis (Goldenseal) root, 48
Hatha Yoga, 185
heat, 166
hemorrhoids, 13
high-velocity/low-amplitude (HVLA), 217
Hyoscyamus niger (henbane), 25
hypnosis, 235

I
incontinence, 15
inositol, 74
interstitial cystitis (IC), 26, 56, 112
irritable bowel syndrome (IBS), 9, 11, 99, 186

K

Kanpo, 5–9
Kegel exercises, 133
kidney stones, 16, 36, 72, 122

L

L-Arginine, 58, 63, 65
L-Citrulline, 66
Levisticum officinale, 36
libido, 13, 137
Lobelia inflata (lobelia), 36
lousewort tincture, 27
low back pain (LBP), 226
low libido, 14, 103
low testosterone, 35
lowered libido, 13

M

maca, 64
maca root (*Lepidium meyenii*),
    70
*Macrotyloma uniflorum var
    uniflorum* (horse gram,
    kulattha), 38
magnesium (Mg), 51, 73
magnolia bark (*Magnolia
    officianlis*), 63
male pelvic pain, 52
male sexual dysfunction, 65
manual feedback, 151
manual lymph drainage, 153
manual therapy, 130
marshmallow, 28
menorrhagia, 12
menstrual irregularities, 10
Mentha x piperita (peppermint),
    38
mixed urinary incontinence, 173

Mucuna pruriens (dopa bean),
    70
muscle energy (ME), 217
myofascial release (MFR), 151,
    217
myofascial trigger point release,
    147

N

Nadi Shodhana, 189
nettle root (*Urtica dioica radix*),
    71
neural mobilization, 149
neuromuscular electrical
    stimulation (NMES), 167

O

obstructive defecation, 176
osteopathy in the cranial field
    (OCF), 218
Oketsu, 7, 10, 14
omega-3 oils: EPA and DHA, 53
omega-3 fatty acid, 102
orgasm dysfunction, 13
osteopathic manipulative
    medicine (OMM), 210
ovarian cysts, 103
overactive bladder (OAB), 25, 49,
    113, 174

P

painful bladder syndrome (PBS),
    16, 56, 93
Panax ginseng (Asian ginseng),
    34, 63
Pausinystalia yohimbe
    (yohimbe), 33
Pedicularis spp (lousewort), 27

pelvic congestion syndrome
(PCS), 153
pelvic floor dyssynergia, 177
pelvic organ prolapse (POP), 134,
206
pelvic pain, 12, 177, 249, 255
PERFECT scheme, 132
peyronie's disease, 34
phimosis, 35
Phyllanthus niuri (chanca
piedra), 37
Piper methysticum (kava) root, 27
Piscidia piscipula (Jamaican
dogwood), 36
pollen extract, 54
polycystic ovarian syndrome
(PCOS), 92, 102
pomegranate, 68
potassium citrate, 73
Pranayama, 187
premature ejaculation (PE), 137,
252
preparation of *Kanpo* herbal
medicine, 17
Probiotics, 56
Prolapse, 137
Prunus africanum (pygeum), 30
psoralea, 57
post-traumatic stress disorder
(PTSD), 228
pubic bone, 213
pudendal nerve, 141
pumpkin seed oil (Cucurbita
maxima), 52
pygeum (*Prunus africana*), 54

Q

Qi, 7, 13
quercetin, 28, 58

R

range of motion (ROM), 139
red reishi, 51
Rehmannia, 57
resveratrol, 67
rhodiola, 67
rhubarb, 57
Rosmarinus officinalis
(rosemary), 38

S

sacroiliac joints, 213
sacrum, 214
Secale cereale (rye) pollen, 28
Serenoa repens (saw palmetto),
28
sexual function, 130, 137
Shang Han Lun, 5
soft tissue mobilization, 148
strain–counterstrain technique,
218
stress incontinence, 26, 59
stress urinary incontinence (SUI),
119, 133, 173
struvite stones, 75

T

Taraxacum officinale
(dandelion), 36
therapeutic ultrasound, 167
Tongkat Ali (*Eurycoma
longifolia*), 70
transcutaneous electrical
stimulation, 167
Tribulus terrestris, 71
Turnera aphrodesiaca, 63
Turnera diffusa (damiana),
33

U

Ujjayi, 189
urge incontinence, 15, 59, 134, 174
urgency, 134
urgency urinary incontinence (UUI), 119
uric acid stones, 74
urinary tract infection (UTI), 15, 20, 46, 110
Urtica dioica (nettle), 23
Urtica dioica (nettle) root, 30

V

Vaccinium macrocarpon (cranberry), 23
vestibulitis, 12

visceral mobilization, 151
vitamin B12, 59
vitamin C, 50, 76
vitamin D, 50
vitamin D deficiency, 110
vitamin D3, 55, 62
vitamin K, 74
vulvar discomfort, 121
vulvar vestibulitis, 177
vulvodynia, 12, 143

Y

Yin yang, 6

Z

zinc, 55, 61, 71

Printed in the United States
By Bookmasters